before using any of the suggested remedies, techniques, or information in this book.

Upon using the information contained in this book, you agree to hold harmless the Author from and against any damages, costs, and expenses, including any legal fees potentially resulting from the application of any of the information provided by this guide. This disclaimer applies to any damages or injury caused by the use and application, whether directly or indirectly, of any advice or information presented, whether for breach of contract, tort, negligence, personal injury, criminal intent, or under any other cause of action.

You agree to accept all risks of using the information presented inside this book. You need to consult a professional medical practitioner in order to ensure you are both able and healthy enough to participate in this program.

Table of Contents

Contents

Introduction

Shift Your Metabolism and Mindset

Let me take you on a short mind trip – the one you've probably heard many times before but the one that needs to be repeated as many times for it to truly stick with you. It's simply a brief overview about the importance of health and how it affects every other aspect of your life.

Your entire existence – your sensory perceptions, your movements, the ideas you have of yourself and the things you do – are the outcries and projections of your consciousness – your consciousness that stems from your body. Everything you feel, do and have flow through your physique to your psyche, which creates the notion of there being a self and a world.

With that being said, I believe it's quite evident that the way you treat your body has a profound impact on your overall well-being and what you're capable of doing. Although the depth of this statement tends to fly past the ear of most people, it's still paramount and should be the focus of our attention.

The fact of the matter is, you can't expect to live a truly fulfilling life and reach your potential as a human being if you suffer from poor health. It's your greatest asset – the one quality that stays with you constantly and keeps echoing in the back of your head, because the state of your physiology quite literally changes the way you perceive and interact with the world.

This corresponds with Maslow's hierarchy of needs as well. The most fundamental needs of any living organism have to do with its physiological necessities, such as survival and reproduction. In that particular order they are: oxygen, water, calories, shelter and sex. Once these are covered, it can begin to think about psychological desires that fall into the camp of socializing, love and group living. Only after that can the organism start thinking about self-actualization – being as great as it can be. This is the playing field, in which you're truly living out your true potential and having peak experiences that allow you to express your creativity, conscience and follow your purpose – it's the sweetest of all truths.

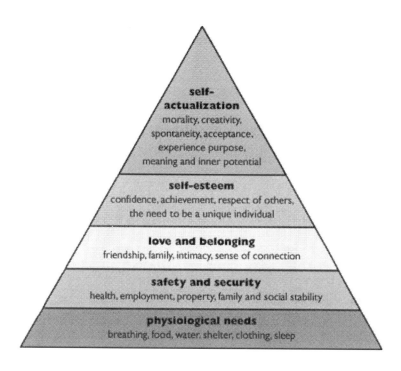

The reason why it's called the hierarchy of needs is that it functions in a hierarchical fashion. Although it may not always be truthful or applicable in a real life context, it's still the perfect directive for us to follow. When it comes to your body, then you have to follow the same progression. You have to start from the bottom and make sure you've laid a solid foundation before you start building anything on top of it, otherwise the entire structure – your entire world construct – will collapse. I want you to take a moment to let that sink in, properly.

What This Book is About:

Now that we've covered the most profound meta-lesson, we've arrived at the purpose of this book. In essence, it's about learning to take care of our body so that we could be healthier, more vibrant and have greater capacity for producing energy, but in its core it's a manual for manipulating our own physiology in a way that would make us stronger, more resilient and efficient.

The two pillar stones of what's written here – the ones that lay the foundation to us achieving optimal health and performance - are two nutritional strategies that have gained a lot of popularity over the past few years, and with a reason. They are Intermittent Fasting (IF) and the Ketogenic Diet (KETO). You will get to know what they are and how they work in the first upcoming chapters. I'm going to delve into the nitty-gritty details of physiology but, don't worry, I'm not going to overwhelm you with too much scientific jargon or concepts that may not find any practical application in your life. Instead, I'll tell you only what you need to know and how you can start using IF and KETO in your life.

But first, let me introduce myself as well. My name is Siim Land – I'm a holistic health practitioner, a writer, a self-

14

experimenter and a high performance coach. In essence, I'm the ultimate creative force of my life, taking action towards living to my full potential while having fun and empowering others at the same time.

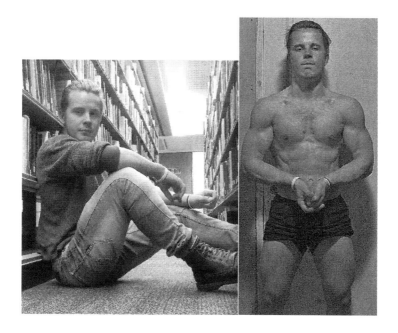

My expertise in IF comes from practicing it for 5-6 years – ever since high school (I'm 22 now). The ketogenic diet found its way into my repertoire in May 2015 and I've been in ketosis – at least in some degree – for nearly 2 years.

I've experimented with these strategies for a long time and I'm always amazed by the sheer effectiveness of them. Every time

I try out a new eating window or make minor adjustments in my nutrition, I discover how much stronger and resilient my body actually is.

By combining IF and keto, I've managed to improve my physical abilities by building purely lean muscle with virtually zero fat gain; enhanced my cognitive performance by making myself mentally sharper and focused; and made myself have an abundance of energy all day every day no matter the time or place. To be honest, I feel Superhuman because I can do what others can't do and say that I'm not capable of doing.

Here's What You Will Learn from This Book:

- Make yourself healthy again
- Improve your biomarkers
- Reverse some of the medical conditions you might have
- Prevent or battle diabetes
- Protect yourself against cancer, tumors and other disease
- Increase your longevity and life-span
- Burn as much fat as you want
- Heal your gut and repair your hormones
- Start building some lean muscle

- Give yourself an abundance of energy

- Always feel satiated and amazing

- Not feel deprived of food or essential nutrients

- Eat delicious food until you're satisfied

Both IF and keto go against a lot of what is considered as healthy or optimal for performance. The villainizing of fat and constant eating has led the majority of the population to becoming obese and diseased. Fortunately, you've found this book and can easily empower your physiology to a much more powerful and efficient state. In my opinion, doing intermittent fasting on a ketogenic diet is the Holy Grail of high performance, longevity and well-being.

The Book is Structured as Follows:

- In Part One, I'm going to teach you the fundamentals of metabolism, nutritional ketosis and fasting. It's the part where we're going to delve into how it works on purely the physiological side. Some of the chapters talk about why you should go on a ketogenic diet, the benefits of fasting and how they can enhance your energy on the mitochondrial level. I'll also step aside from pure science for a moment and rant about The Breakfast Myth and how fasting can make you free.

- Part Two is about the HOW – how to get into ketosis, how to know whether or not you're in, how to choose your type of fasting and how to fast and feast. I'm also going to give you the guidelines on how to fast for several days in a row and how to use exogenous ketones.

- Part Three takes everything what you've learned and puts it all together – it's about combining IF and keto. I'm going to tell you what changes you should make and what are the best foods to buy on a ketogenic diet. Because I not only want to empower your physiology but your psychology as well, I'll give you some advice on creating new ketogenic habits. Eventually, I'll provide you with a four-phase adaptation blueprint that will help you to get used to the ketogenic diet and start practicing extended fasting. Most importantly, there's a separate chapter covering all of the mistakes you could make and how to avoid them. Lastly, there's also room for some recipes (in a fasting book?!) and supplementation.

Using Keto Fasting is, first and foremost, a tool to empower how you feel, how you perform, the state of your health and what you can accomplish. There are several ways you can structure your own eating strategy because IF and keto simply allow you incredible metabolic flexibility. The core essence of it is that you'll become an incredibly efficient at your own bioenergetics production and capable of being the Superhuman you know you can be.

Part One

Creating a Metabolic Advantage

This part is structured as follows:

- Chapter One – Metabolic Crash Course
  - What are Calories and How Many Should You Consume
  - Most Important Hormones
  - Fat Storage and Loss Explained
  - Why 'Eat Less and Move More' Doesn't Work
- Chapter Two – What is Ketosis
  - Indigenous Ketogenic Societies
  - Is Ketosis Safe
- Chapter Three – Why Go on a Ketogenic Diet
  - Ketosis for Health
  - Athletes Going Against the Grain
  - Keto Smart
  - Why Fructose Isn't Good
  - Keto Sleep
- Chapter Four – Enter the Fasting Fray
  - The Physiology of Fasting

There's a ton of value I'm giving you already, but don't worry, there's more to come in the subsequent parts. This is just the beginning, so let us begin.

Chapter One

Metabolic Crash Course

This book also includes a lot of the basic knowledge about nutrition and optimal health in general. For long term results, you want to actually understand what we're talking about here, otherwise you'll be simply implementing a quick-fix that will leave you vulnerable for future mistakes.

The reason why 80% of diets fail is that the people don't learn from their mistakes. They have no clue about what causes their obesity and what to do about it. Instead of getting to the root cause of their condition - which is their ignorance - they are focusing on the symptoms – their poor body composition and medical condition. This makes it too easy to fall into the trap of starting to blame the society, their ancestral "fat" genes or lack of willpower.

Simply telling you what to eat won't give you the solution to your problems. You'll do great for a while – you'll lose some weight and even regain some of your lost vigor. However, it will only work until it doesn't. When that happens, you'll be dumbstruck, trying to figure out what went wrong. You then give up all hope and return to your old habits.

Eating random things without knowing what further effect it has on your metabolism is the worst mindset to have. Remember, the state of your physiology has profound effects on every other aspect of your life as well. There needs to also be a change in your overall mentality and understanding of food. Once you have an understanding of the basics, you'll be able to always know the reason as to why you feel in a certain way at any given time.

Rather than fixing symptoms, I would prefer going to the root cause of the issue, which is ignorance about optimal nutrition and healthy living. That's why I'm going to give you a brief metabolic crash course about the most relevant and essential definitions and principles that you need to understand.

Don't worry, I'm not going to get too in over our heads and will keep it as easy to comprehend as possible. As Einstein put it: *"Everything should be made as simple as possible, but not simpler."* I could explain this to a child, but there needs to be some input from your part as well. This is invaluable knowledge of life, especially in our modern environment, and should be taught at schools.

Let's Start from Ground Zero

- **Calories.** A calorie is a unit of energy that produce heat. In the context of nutrition, they are a measure of the amount of energy in food and liquids. Within the body, they're used as fuel to produce the necessary energy we need to survive. By burning off what we consume we provide ourselves with a source of power that allows us to function. There is a certain amount of calories any given organism needs, which is dependent of how much heat has to be produced for maintenance.

The first law of thermodynamics states that: *"the change in internal energy of a system is equal to the heat added to the system minus the work done by the system."*

What it says is that weight loss or gain is controlled by the inner energy balance. The body will always try to maintain an inner state of equilibrium called *'homeostasis.'* Calories in versus calories out determine body composition. Basically, you can eat whatever you want and lose fat, as long as you stay at a negative energy balance.

However, weight loss doesn't necessarily equal fat loss. Nutrition influences our hormones, which have a much more profound impact on our health and longevity. You don't want to damage your organs or waste valuable muscle tissue in the process. Looking good on the outside does not mean that everything is well on the inside.

How Many Calories Should You Eat?

Well, it would depend on your total daily energy expenditure (TDEE). This includes your basal metabolic rate (BMR) and activity levels.

Use these simple formulas to calculate your basal metabolic rate (BMR). This is the number which we would have to consume by doing nothing – simply breathing and lying in bed.

- **Imperial system.**

   o Women: BMR=655 + (4.35 x weight in pounds) + (4.7 x height in inches) - (4.7 x age in years)

- Men: BMR = 66 + (6.23 x weight in pounds) + (12.7 x height in inches) - (6.8 x age in year)

- **Metric system.**

  - Women: BMR = 655 + (9.6 x weight in kilos) + (1.8 x height in cm) - (4.7 x age in years)

  - Men: BMR = 66 + (13.7 x weight in kilos) + (5 x height in cm) - (6.8 x age in years)

What adds onto it are our activity levels - how much we move around, how often and at what intensity. That's why an athlete needs more calories than a sedentary person would because they're constantly using energy. Don't start basing your daily intake on step-counters or what Fitbit watches tell you. Instead, start paying more attention to how much you're eating and see how it influences your weight.

Make your adjustments according to your current physique goals. If you want to gain muscle, then add a small surplus of about 200-500 calories. To lose fat, eat less, about a 500 calorie deficit.

You don't have to weigh your food either. Small changes in grams and percentages are insignificant. When on the ketogenic diet you have to pay even less attention to this, as the foods you eat are very satiating and prevent you from getting fat easily. What's more, with intermittent fasting it's quite difficult to overeat because of the restricted feeding window.

You would need to pay attention to calories only during the initial adaptation period when your body is still getting used to its new fuel source. However, you should still educate yourself about the caloric values and macronutrient proportions of all foods. This way you'll know what effect food has on you and can base your intake exactly on what you need or desire.

Buy an ordinary food scale and start tracking your food intake for about a week or two. This will help you understand how many calories and in what proportions you're consuming. It's necessary for you to remember the approximate values of those numbers so that you could always optimize your intake by heart.

Use the online app called MyFitnessPal to log your food intake. It's free and super easy to use.

After a while, you don't have to pay any more attention to this. You'll know it by heart and can easily guesstimate how much energy is packed in all foods. It's like a superpower – cyclops sight. We should all have this knowledge about nutrition.

Moving on.

- **Metabolism.** The word comes from Greek and means "change" which in the context of our body is the transformation of cells, digestion and transportation of nutrients. Basically, the furnace of our organism which governs energy transmission and usage. It's divided into catabolism, breakdown of tissue, and anabolism, building up. Throughout the day we're constantly moving between the two. After we eat, we begin to use that food for growth and repair. Once a few hours have passed, or while sleeping, we begin to rely on our own storage and use that for fuel.

Calories, however, are not all equal and are divided into 3 macronutrients which make up the nutritional quality of any given food.

- **Proteins and amino acids.** These are the building blocks of our organism. They are the structural framework of all cells that give them form. Our muscles, skin, hair, nails, organs, bones are all made out of protein. Amino acids are necessary for cellular energy metabolism and anabolic tissue repair and enhancement. The richest sources of protein are meat, eggs, fish but it can also be found in nuts, seeds and to a much lesser degree in vegetables, legumes and beans. In 1 gram of protein there are 4 calories.

- **Lipids and fats.** They are also known as triglycerides which are 3 long chains of fatty acids. Their function is to govern metabolic, hormonal and structural processes. They are divided into saturated, monounsaturated, polyunsaturated and trans fats, which depends on the amount of bonding of the carbon atoms in the chain. Some of them are essential - such as omega-3's and omega-6's -

because they cannot be synthesized within the body itself. In food, the purest sources of only fats are all types of oils, butter, lard, ghee etc. but they can also be found in nuts, cheese, heavy cream, meat, eggs and fish. If our energy balance is positive, we will convert these nutrients into triglycerides and store them in our adipose tissue, or, in more earthly terms, our body fat. Once in the negative, we take those same lipids and use them for energy. In 1 gram of fat there are 9 calories.

- **Carbohydrates.** The main energy source of the body which are basically sugars. Their role is to fuel our activities and they can be stored within the body as glycogen, in the liver 100-150 grams worth and in the muscle cells for up to 500 grams. They're divided into galactose (milk sugars), fructose (fruit, such as apples, grapes, oranges etc.) and glucose (mainly starchy vegetables, tubers, like potatoes, and grains, such as wheat and rice). Consumption of carbohydrates influences our blood sugar and depends upon the glycemic index/load of a given food. If there isn't not much fiber content or other macronutrients to slow down the digestion, then simple sugars will raise blood sugar quite rapidly. Fiber is the indigestible part of a plant that passes through our gut mostly intact. It's beneficial for digestion and feeds the good gut microbiome. In 1 gram of carbohydrates there are 4 calories.

- **Micronutrients.** What governs the macros are the vitamins, minerals and enzymes of any given food. They're equally as important for overall health and wellbeing. Calories in calories out is mainly responsible for body composition but for high end performance we want to get as much actual benefits from what we eat as possible. Nutrient dense food will give us more energy and yield better results. Because our body can't produce micronutrients by itself, they need to be derived from diet. Unfortunately, not all food is equal in terms of micronutrient ratios. For us to function like a well-oiled machine and get the most bang for our buck, we need to either eat quality food or supplement our deficiencies about which I will talk about in the coming chapters.

The Most Important Hormones

There are also some very important hormones that we need to know about.

- **Insulin** is the key hormone when it comes to the storage and distribution of nutrients within the body. If it's elevated, then we are more prone to store the food we eat whether into fat or muscle cells. When it's low we start to rely more on our own adipose tissue for fuel. Insulin gets released by the pancreas in response to the rise of blood sugar and tries to bring it back to normal to prevent hyperglycemia (too high blood sugar levels) or hypoglycemia (too low). It's most significantly caused by the consumption of high-glycemic carbohydrates, very little by protein or fibrous vegetables and not at all by fat. In the case of insulin sensitivity, we're quite efficient with regulating this hormone and don't need a lot to shuttle nutrients into our cells. If we're resistant, however, we can't bring it back down and we'll have constantly elevated levels of it, which can lead to obesity, diabetes and cardiovascular disease.

- **Leptin** regulates the feeling of satiety and hunger. Its role is to signal our brain to eat to prevent starvation. However, if we're resistant to it then the lines of communication will be cut short and our mind will never get the information that the body has received enough calories. In that case, your body is satisfied but your brain is still starving and keeps on craving for more food. It usually goes hand in hand with insulin resistance, as they both are caused by the consumption of simple carbohydrates and sugar with a lot of fat at the same time.

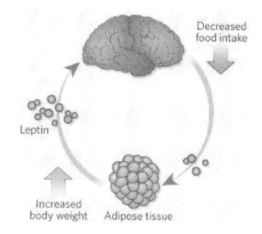

- **Ghrelin** is the hormone that creates hunger in the first place. It gets released when our stomach is empty, indicating that it wants to eat something.

- **Glucagon** is the counterpart of insulin and also gets produced by the pancreas. It gets released when the concentration of glucose in the blood stream gets too low. The liver then starts to convert stored glycogen into glucose and increase fatty acid utilization.

- **Serotonin** is a neurotransmitter primarily found in the gastrointestinal tract and the central nervous system (CNS) of animals. It's also considered to be the relaxation hormone which contributes to the feeling of well-being and happiness. Proteins contain an amino acid called tryptophan that gets converted into serotonin in the brain. Carbohydrates can also release serotonin.

- **Human growth hormone (HGH)** stimulates growth and cell development within the body. Its role is to produce and regenerate the organism's tissue and has anabolic effects because it raises the concentration of glucose and free fatty acids in the blood stream. Children have a lot of growth hormone because they're constantly growing. For adults, HGH increases muscle building and fat burning. It's the Holy Grail Hormone of longevity, high end performance and excellent body composition.

- **Insulin-like growth factor (IGF-1)** is a hormone that plays a crucial part in childhood growth and also has anabolic effects in adults as well. It's one of the most effective natural activators of pathways responsible for cellular growth and an inhibitor of cellular death. IGF-1 is closely connected with HGH. The release of HGH into the blood stream by the anterior pituitary gland also stimulates the liver to produce IGF-1 which causes systemic growth in almost every cell in the body, especially muscle, cartilage, bone, liver, kidney, nerves, skin and lungs. It can also nerve cell growth and development. Currently research is not clear about whether or not IGF-1 signaling is positively or negatively associated with aging and cancer. Over-expression may lead to cancer but on the other hand natural enhanced actions of HGH and IGF-1 are effective ways of establishing an anabolic state, supporting the immune system.

GROWTH HORMONE

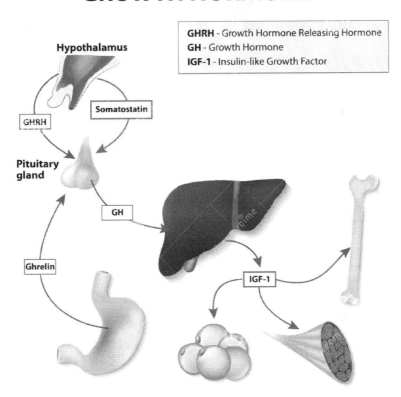

> **GHRH** - Growth Hormone Releasing Hormone
> **GH** - Growth Hormone
> **IGF-1** - Insulin-like Growth Factor

- **Testosterone (T-Force)** is associated with masculine behavior but it's also found in women as well. This is yet another anabolic hormone that enhances muscle building, increases strength and torches fat burning, but it also has some cognitive benefits. Too low levels of testosterone will decrease reproductive functions, cause fat storage and increase risk of cardiovascular disease. The best T-boosters are heavy resistance training, high intensity interval training (HIIT), dietary fat intake and proper sleep. Maintaining a straight posture and not slumping over will also release testosterone because of the powerful feeling and confidence we get. The connection between our physiology and psychology is especially clear here. Our mind can affect the body's biochemistry and *vice versa*.

- **Cortisol,** also known as the main stress and *"fight or flight"* hormone, controls our energy in strenuous circumstances. It's the counterpart of testosterone. Evolutionarily, its role is to enable us to survive in situations of life and death. It gets elevated when we would have to run away from a lion, fight off a pack of wolves, while drowning or chasing after dinner. As a result, glycogen and norepinephrine get released into the blood stream to provide more energy for the muscles. The body perceives every type of stress response as the same and sitting in traffic, being nervous about public speaking, exercising hard or arguing with someone release as much cortisol as fighting a tiger would. Occasional short spikes of stress are necessary and can be beneficial as it conditions us to handle difficult situations – a phenomenon called 'hormesis,' which we will be talking about in a later chapter. If cortisol remains elevated for too long, then anabolism and catabolism get out of balance, leading to decreased levels of testosterone and excessive breakdown of tissue.

- **Norepinephrine** (NE) or noradrenaline (NA) functions in the brain as a hormone and neurotransmitter. Outside of the brain, norepinephrine gets released into the blood stream by the adrenal glands. This is supposed to help the body mobilize itself into action during fight or flight situations. It promotes arousal, alertness, vigilance, enhances focus and increases heart rate. As glucose gets released, more blood will also flow into skeletal muscle. However, this happens at the expense of reducing blood flow to the gastrointestinal track – once you go into fight or flight your digestion stops.

These hormones get released within us in response to the food we eat, what we do, our current condition, degree of sensitivity to them and also the time of the day (circadian rhythms). This means that we're totally in control of our own biology and can influence how they affect us and when.

Fat Storage and Loss

How do we store fat? Or a much better question would be to ask, why do we get fat in the first place? In an evolutionarily unforgiving environment *i.e.* the savannah it was essential for early humans (any living organism really) to have a solution for surviving times of scarcity. Being such energy dependent creatures as we are, simply flipping it and starving to death, when we run out of food, would not benefit our chances at natural selection. Instead of wasting away, our body has developed a complex set of mechanisms that allow it to maintain its functioning and actually increase the rate of it.

You might think that it would be so much better if we didn't get fat – everyone would simply look like fitness models and we wouldn't have to think about eating. However, that is yet another attempt to apply a quick-fix solution.

We need to store fat so that we would have a back-up supply when *'sh#t hits the fan'* (SHTF). What's more important, simply carrying around pounds of extra calories with us is useless, even detrimental, if the body doesn't know how to convert it back into energy. That's why it's so important to practice IF and keto even in a society where food is abundant.

Fat Storage 101

Lipogenesis is the process by which acetyl-CoA (a molecule that partakes in metabolizing calories) gets converted to fatty acids. Our adipose tissue stores fat in the form of triglycerides into *'adipocytes'* (fat cells). What it basically means is that, if you're eating above your needed caloric balance, then food molecules (whether that be carbs, fat or protein) need to be converted into triglycerides before they can be stored in the adipose tissue. Our carbohydrate stores are limited to our liver and muscle glycogen (100-150 grams + 300-500 grams); and we can't store protein endogenously; but our fat stores are potentially limitless.

How Fat Burning Takes Place

To melt fat off your body, you have to first *"release"* it. This happens by a process called *'lipolysis,'* which breaks down those very triglycerides we previously stored into glycerol and free fatty acids (FFAs).

Lipolysis gets triggered by the following hormones: glucagon, norepinephrine, ghrelin, growth hormone, testosterone, and cortisol.

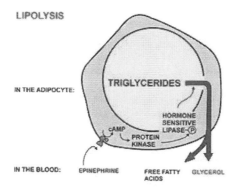

Glucagon is the counterpart of insulin that rises when our blood sugar levels are low. It makes the liver convert stored glycogen into glucose and increase FFA utilization.

Why Eat Less Move More Doesn't Work

The reason is that, it's based on a false idea about how our bodies work and use calories. It looks at it as if all calories were equal in terms of nutritional value and the way they get metabolized. This is the *"calories in versus calories out"* type of approach that is completely false and could work only in our wildest dreams.

The real situation is this: our body uses two distinct ways to store energy in the body. They are carbohydrates in the form of glycogen and triglycerides as body fat.

There's also a huge difference between 100 calories from let's say broccoli and 100 calories from a candy bar because they get metabolized differently.

Weight loss plateaus occur because of homeostasis - the body adapts to the new conditions. If you maintain a reduced caloric intake for some time, then your metabolism declines to match the reduced intake. As a result, you reach a new set point of caloric balance and need to decrease it again to keep making progress.

The key hormone when it comes to body composition is insulin, which regulates the storage and distribution of nutrients. If it's constantly elevated, then we won't be able to burn fat and will actually be more prone to depositing it. That is why we would want to keep it low for the majority of the day. If you want to lose fat, then from a physiological perspective, it doesn't make sense to eat high-carb meals several times per day.

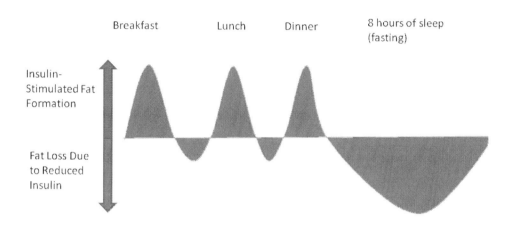

Insulin gets released in response to rising blood sugar levels so that it could bring it down to normal. This happens most by consuming high amounts of carbohydrates, very little by lean protein and not at all by fat.

High carb diets make '*lipase*' - the enzyme involved in breaking down body fat - almost completely inactive. By triggering insulin, you put a harsh stop to burning fat for the rest of the day and possibly even the next one to come.

Therefore, the secret to melting off body fat is to keep insulin levels low and restrict carbohydrate intake.

The ability to melt off fat is a unique skill to have and a very handy one in our toolkit. It's not about weight loss, but more like simply being an efficient fat burner. The differentiating factor from burning sugar is that you'll be using your own adipose tissue to create energy and you'll be making more of it.

What Happens When Glucose Runs Out

When your liver glycogen stores get depleted, you increase glucagon and lipolysis by starting to produce more ketone bodies. After a while, you enter a state of nutritional ketosis, in which your body uses fat for fuel, instead of glucose. This can happen after fasting for 2-3 days or following a well-formulated ketogenic diet for several weeks.

When in ketosis, you literally will be taking the cells from your own belly fat and converting it into energy. For that to happen you would still need to be in a negative energy balance, but this is so easy to induce on a ketogenic diet.

High carb low fat diets with not a lot of fiber can lead to leptin resistance. You can eat copious amounts of sugar without even feeling like you've consumed anything. It's so easy to gorge yourself and not notice how much you've eaten. The signal that you've received enough calories disappears into the void and gets silenced by your subconscious mind whose motivations urge you to keep on eating. Now, eat a tablespoon of salted butter or coconut oil and you won't get any cravings whatsoever. You'll light up your taste buds but won't enter this vicious cycle of wanting more. Fat feeds your brain and keeps your body well-nourished.

Eating fat triggers a hormone called 'cholecystokinin' (CKK), which tells your body you're full. It gives the brain immense amounts of long lasting energy and keeps it satiated.

Although I think that most people would benefit greatly from lowering their carbohydrate intake at least to some degree, not everyone is interested in following a ketogenic diet. That's perfectly fine, as long as you still stick to a whole foods based diet 80% of the time. However, by you picking up this book in particular, you're more than eager to try it out. That's what we will turn to next, which is the nitty-gritty of ketosis and what physiological effects it causes.

Chapter Takeaway:

- The first principle of energy balance and weight loss is "calories in vs calories out."
- However, a much more important factor is the hormonal and metabolic response to what was eaten.
- Insulin is the most important hormone when it comes to maintaining a healthy body composition.
- We would want to keep this highly anabolic hormone low for the majority of the time.

Chapter Two

What is Ketosis

The human body is a complex system that can adapt to almost anything. It has found a solution to solving the bioenergetics component of being self-sufficient and resourceful. Ketosis is just that – an irreplaceable part of our biology that creates *endogenous* (from within) energy.

In a nutshell, ketosis is a metabolic state in which the body has shifted from using glucose as the primary fuel source into supplying its energy demands with ketone bodies.

This happens when the liver glycogen stores are depleted and a substitute is necessary for the brain to maintain its functioning.

Both carbohydrates and fats can be used for the production of energy, but they're different in quality. However, in the presence of both, the body will always prefer the former because sugar can be easily accessed and quickly absorbed. To get the most out of the latter, there needs to be a period of keto-adaptation. The length of it depends on how reliant you are of glucose and how well your body accepts this new fuel source.

Ketosis is an altered, but still natural, metabolic state that occurs either over a prolonged period of fasting or by restricting carbohydrate intake significantly, usually up to less than 50 grams per day [i].

After an overnight's fast already, our liver glycogen stores will be depleted and *Captain Liver* starts to produce more ketone bodies. This, in return, will increase the availability of fatty acids in the blood stream, which the body then begins to utilize for the production of energy. It can be derived from both food and the adipose tissue.

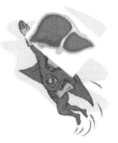

Captain Liver
to the Rescue.

This process is called 'beta-oxidation'. When fat is broken down by the liver, glycerol and fatty acid molecules are released. The fatty acid gets broken down even more through *'ketogenesis'* that produces a ketone body called 'acetoacetate'. This is then converted further into two other type of ketone bodies. (1) *'Beta-hydroxybutyrate'* (BHB), which is the preferred fuel source for the brain and (2) *'acetone'*, that can be metabolized into glucose, but is mainly excreted as waste.

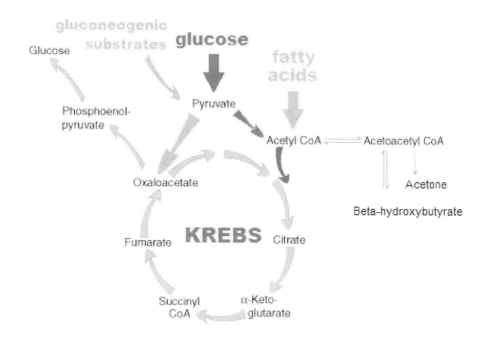

When you're running on glucose you go down the pathway of *'glycolysis'* and create *'pyruvate'*. All of these molecules get burned inside the mitochondria and <u>you can get 25% more energy from using beta-hydroxybutyrate</u> as fuel. In this scenario of fat utilization, we're taking the more efficient route that increases the density of our cellular power plants.

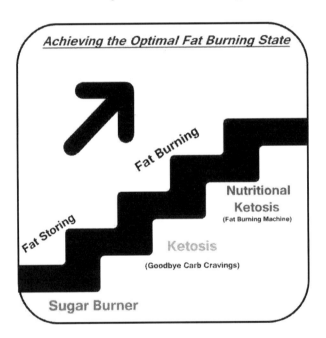

Nutritional ketosis is not the same as *'ketoacidosis'*, which causes the pH levels in the blood to drop and become acidic. This can result with a coma and eventually death. Usually, the body manages to maintain the acidity of the blood within a normal range despite the presence of ketones. Ketoacidosis occurs mostly with type-1 diabetes and excessive alcohol consumption.

After the initial period of adaptation, the body's biochemistry will be completely altered. Approximately 75% of the energy used by the brain will be provided by ketones and the liver will change its enzymes from dominantly digesting carbohydrates to actually preferring fat[ii]. Protein catabolism decreases significantly, as fat stores are mobilized and the use of ketones increases. Muscle glycogen gets used even less and the majority of our caloric demands will be derived from the adipose tissue.

Nutritional ketosis is perfectly safe and a great metabolic state to be in. This process is an adaptive response and completely normal. During periods of famine it will enable us to survive and maintain our vitality. If the body doesn't know how to use its stored fat for fuel, it would perish, once it runs out of sugar.

Indigenous Ketogenic Societies

Over the course of history, most aboriginal tribes have subsisted solely on high fat diets. In environments where there aren't many plants to be found, people rely primarily on meat.

The Innuit and Eskimos have lived off whale blubber, seal meat, salmon, cheese and caribou for centuries. Fat is their most precious commodity, as it gives them the extra calories they need to survive in such harsh climate. In fact, rent on land in some places is paid with butter. Despite that high amount of saturated fat and cholesterol in their diet, heart disease, diabetes and cancer were largely unknown during their aboriginal era. Only after they came in contact with white man's white refined carbohydrates did other diseases of the civilization catch up with them and they got obese.

The Masai tribe in Africa also follows a ketogenic diet. They're pastoralists and subsist mainly on their cattle, by eating their meat, drinking their unpasteurized milk and raw blood. Masai warriors are definitely a lot healthier and fitter than the majority of the people in our society.

Even in the Western world there are nations who eat a ton of fat. The Mediterranean Diet is thought to be the healthiest of them all. It consists of mainly fish, olive oil, cheese and vegetables. People from this region have less heart disease and better blood markers. Researchers from the States figured that it had to do with the low amount of saturated fat and cholesterol in their food. However, the Greek Orthodox Church also preaches a lot of fasting, which has even more profound health benefits. In fact, the more religious folk fast more than 200 days a year. This is the real cause for their vitality. As this ancient healing practice gets less popular amongst young people, disease begins to rise again because there are still a lot of refined grains and carbohydrates in the diet, such as pasta, bread and pizza.

Is Ketosis Safe

One fear that some physicians have about the ketogenic diet is that it can't sustain healthy functioning of an organism. How will your body and brain survive if there are no carbohydrates? Let me explain.

An essential nutrient is something that's required for normal physiological functioning and the survival of the organism[iii]. It cannot be synthesized by the body and thus has to be obtained from a dietary source. <u>Carbohydrates are non-essential, unlike amino acids and fatty acids,</u> which we don't actually need to live and can function very well without.

Amino acids and fat are essential building blocks of all the cells in our body. Protein is used to create new muscle tissue, whereas the lipids balance our hormones that instigate these processes in the first place and protect cell membrane.

Why Do We Have to Eat So Much?

The biggest reason why we have to consume so many calories every single day is to feed our hungry brain. It comprises less than 5% of our body weight but demands about 20% of our total energy expenditure. To maintain stable blood sugar levels and a caloric balance, it needs to have access to fuel all of the time.

The brain can use only about 120 grams of glucose a day [iv], which means you still need at least 30 grams of glucose while running on max ketones. That doesn't mean it ought to come from dietary carbohydrates.

During a process called '*gluconeogenesis*' (creation of new sugar), the liver converts amino acids found in food and glycerol, which is the backbone of triglycerides, into glucose. While in a deep fasted state, glycerol can contribute up to 21.6% of glucose production[v]. It's estimated that about 200 grams of glucose can be manufactured daily by the liver and kidneys from dietary protein and fat intake [vi]. That's more than enough.

Once you keto-adapt, your body and brain won't even need that much glucose, as they will happily use ketones instead. Carbohydrates are the default fuel source but not because they're better than fatty acids by any means. The body simply prefers them because sugar is easy to store and quick to absorb.

However, the brain is made up of 60% fat and runs a lot better on ketones. In fact, the high amounts of fat found in animal products and meat were probably one of the driving forces of our increased brain size. By eating solely plant foods, we wouldn't have managed to get enough excess energy for our neural network to improve itself.

In ketosis, the brain begins to use less glucose and the small amount it needs can be derived from ketogenic foods. Muscles begin to release less glycogen as well and the entire body starts using ketones for fuel. It makes the entire organism more efficient and powerful. If that doesn't give you a big enough of a reason as to why you should do the ketogenic diet, then the next chapter probably will.

Chapter Takeaway

- Ketosis is a distinctive, yet perfectly natural and healthy, metabolic state, in which the body has shifted from using glucose as its primary fuel source into creating energy from fatty acids and ketone bodies.
- Ketosis occurs either over fasting for several days or following a well-formulated ketogenic diet for a few weeks.
- Ketosis is not the same as ketoacidosis and is perfectly healthy.
- Carbohydrates aren't needed for the healthy functioning of an organism.
- When in ketosis, the brain derives 75% of its energy demands from ketone bodies and the body begins to need less overall glycogen.

Chapter Three

Why Go on a Ketogenic Diet

Hopefully, you're beginning to see the slowly emerging advantages of ketosis. In comparison to the recommended dietary pyramid, the ketogenic diet looks very appealing. There are a lot of health benefits to this, covering both physical and mental aspects.

Advantages of Ketosis

The most obvious advantage is increased fat oxidation[vii]. Consuming carbohydrates will make our body secrete more insulin. When this hormone is elevated we're more prone to storing rather than burning. If it's constantly high, we'll never be able to actually tap into using our own resources.

The by-products of glucose metabolism are '*advanced glycation end-products*' (AGEs), which promote inflammation and oxidative stress[viiiix], by binding a protein or lipid molecule with sugar. They speed up aging[x], and can cause diabetes. This doesn't happen when burning clean fuel - good quality fat. Also, the constantly elevated levels of circulating blood sugar are associated with nerve malfunctioning, high morbidity, bacterial infection, cancer progression and Alzheimer's. Carbs aren't necessarily the devil, but more and more research is pointing towards the dangers of consuming refined carbohydrates.

The #1 food for tumors is sugar. Eating keto foods, prevents the accumulation of excess glucose in the blood, which hypothetically could lead to the cellular suicide of cancer. With no carbohydrates for it to feed upon, it will potentially disappear completely, at least it will diminish in size. At the same time, your healthy cells will still be nourished because they'll be using fat for fuel.

Ketosis reduces natural hunger to a bare minimum and regulates appetite[xi]. This is the result of the body being able to generate energy from both the adipose tissue and dietary fat intake. The ability to go without meals for 24 hours and more, while not suffering any stomach pains or carb driven cravings of insanity, is incredibly empowering, not to mention useful for both fitness and reducing fat composition.

Our body is made to burn fat. The adipose tissue is like a black hole with infinite storage capacity. Any surplus calorie we don't need right away gets deposited for future use. When in ketosis, we'll be withdrawing energy from our own body fat to maintain a caloric balance.

Ketones are the *"superfuel"* reigning supreme over both glucose and free fatty acids. As you can remember, they can produce 25% more energy and will cover 75% of the brains energy demands. When in ketosis, you begin to need less and less glucose, which makes your biology more and more self-sufficient.

Ketosis for Health

Because of the fact that a fat molecule has twice the amount of calories than a carbohydrate one it gets digested a lot slower. **Unlike sugar, that gets burned up easily, ketones move steadily and provide long lasting energy.**

This also prevents any rise in blood sugar from taking place, which happens after consuming something with a high glycemic index. Instant bursts of energy will inevitably fall as quickly. What goes up must come down. This results in hypoglycemia (a crash of blood sugar) and sleepiness. With fat that doesn't happen, as we will have an abundant fuel source, thus always feeling great. Instead of secreting insulin and taking our bodies for a rollercoaster ride, we maintain a steady stream of energy.

Following a low carbohydrate high fat diet has been proven very effective against a lot of the chronic illnesses people struggle with.

- Reduction in triglycerides[xii]
- Increase in HDL cholesterol (the good one)[xiii]
- Drop in blood pressure[xiv] and insulin levels[xv]

All of which prevent heart disease, diabetes and metabolic syndrome[xvi]. For optimal health it looks very appealing.

Athletes Going Against the Grain (Pun Intended)

If you're physically active and fit, then you probably don't have to worry about obesity and other ailments. However, this doesn't mean that you can't pick up any disease or develop a severe medical condition.

Insulin resistance happens in the case of consuming too many simple carbohydrates and being constantly on a blood sugar rollercoaster ride. Even the most athletic of individuals can become diabetic and a lot of professional athletes already have.

Following a low carb diet, while still training, ought to optimize our health first and foremost. However, there are also a lot of performance enhancing benefits to using fat for fuel.

The Advantages of Fat as Fuel

The maximum amount of glucose our bodies can store is about 2000 calories (approximately 400-500 grams of carbohydrates in the muscles, 100-150 grams in the liver and about 15 grams in the blood). Once that runs out, more fatty acids are produced to supply the demand. Although this is the point in which adipose tissue is being used it only happens to a certain degree. To still get some form of glucose, the body will also begin to break down a bit of the protein in muscles and organs to create sugar. The reason is that it's not that adapted to primarily using ketones. To prevent this from happening, a person would need to be constantly adding in more carbohydrates to fuel their activities.

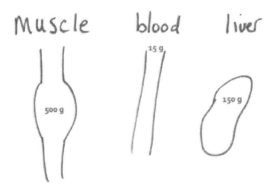

In ketosis, however, the main source of energy is significantly bigger. **Even the leanest of people with 7% body fat carry around more than 20 000 calories with them at all times.** Re-feeding isn't necessary as there is always some fuel available. This also preserves muscles and other vital organs from being catabolized. Instead of being a quick sugar burner, we can become efficient fat burners instead after we keto-adapt.

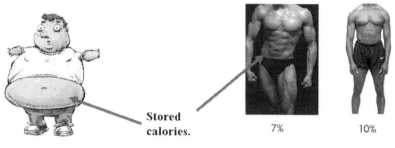

Stored calories.

7%   10%

20 000 -30 000 calories

Ketogenic dieting is becoming very popular amongst endurance athletes, especially ultra-runners and ironman triathletes who have to perform at a high level for extreme durations. By carrying around their own fuel on their bodies they can tap into an abundance of energy. They literally go against the grain of everything in optimal sport's nutrition.

For instance, Sami Inkinen and his wife Meredith Loring rowed across the Pacific Ocean from California to Hawaii in 45 days, while following a low-carb, sugar-free, high-fat ketogenic diet. Despite being physically active for 21 hours a day, they did not suffer any decrease in performance, health or cravings for carbs. Such adaptation shows that we are capable of a lot more than we actually think. How else did our ancestors complete their epic journeys of exploration and migration across the globe?

In a study on advanced triathletes, the group who followed a ketogenic approach instead of the traditional high-carb diet showed 2-3 times higher peak fat oxidation during submaximal exercise[xvii].

Contrary to popular belief physical performance does not suffer by ditching the carbs. It is also used in strength sports such as powerlifting and gymnastics[xviii] where the intensities are lot higher. Bodybuilders use periods of low-carb eating to prepare for shows and improve body composition. If you haven't already, then you should also check out my book for low carb strength athletes called Keto Bodybuilding. There is some overlap regarding ketosis but it also includes a ton of knowledge about the physiology of building muscle and resistance training.

In my own experience, I haven't noticed any negative side-effects of ketosis after proper adaptation. I have managed to improve every aspect of my training and health. It definitely feels great and is well worth the effort.

Keto Smart

In addition to performance oriented benefits, ketosis also has cognitive and mental ones. There's a big difference between being high on keto versus sugar.

Because of how evolutionarily valuable glucose is, the brain's reward endorphin system lights up every time we consume it, motivating us to want more. We release a lot of the "feel-good" chemicals, such as dopamine and serotonin. Cravings and hunger pains come from some people's mind kicking into overdrive and losing their reason over something sweet.

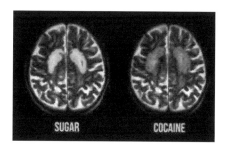

As you can see from this picture, the brain's reward system lights up the same way on sugar as it does on hard drugs. In neurological terms, binge eating and drug addiction are the same thing[xix].

This happens so that we would be motivated to repeat our actions in the future. Our taste buds are designed to recognize sweetness and fire up every single time. Feeling good after eating something sugary puts us on a short high and makes us want more.

Sugar cravings are caused by an energy crisis in the body. If the brain doesn't get access to fuel, it will try to motivate you to find something to eat. Because, by default, it only knows how to use glucose, it will also expect to have it.

However, if you've plugged into your largest fuel tank - your own body fat - then you won't experience these cravings. That's why people lose their sweet tooth completely when on a low carb diet. Their body detoxifies itself from sugar and the mind will get clearer.

Sugar doesn't actually provide us with that much energy and is mainly an illusion. It's a way of trapping our own ATP production. We might have a lot of stored calories but we won't be able to access them, because of inactive hormone sensitive-lipase. This leads to *mental bonking* and *physical exhaustion* in everything you do, whether that be training, reading or anything else. That's why it's important to go through keto adaptation to teach the body how to use fat for fuel.

By avoiding carbohydrates, we also avoid the ups and downs of blood sugar, thus allowing our brain to function properly. By having a steady stream of energy, it doesn't have to be on the lookout for glucose. Some is indeed needed, which gets created by the liver, but the majority can be derived from ketones.

With the brain satisfied, our cognition has the opportunity to flourish. This allows us to maintain mental clarity and avoid mind fog, which accompanies the consumption of whole grains and processed carbohydrates.

Why Fructose Isn't Good

Fructose can only be metabolized by the liver and can't be used as muscle glycogen. It therefore is completely useless to the body. In high amounts it actually becomes toxic because of the liver having to work extra hard to get rid of it.

Excess fructose can damage the liver and cause insulin resistance, which means pancreas can't pump out enough insulin to lower your blood sugar. This is a precursor to diabetes, as sugar will flood your blood stream for longer and cause more damage to the blood vessels.

Fructose can also cause rapid leptin resistance. Leptin controls your appetite and metabolism. If you're resistant, then you'll gain weight easily and can't stop gorging yourself.

The reaction of fructose with proteins is 7 times higher than with glucose. Because of that, AGEs get produced at an even greater rate. While your body can't use fructose as energy, the bad bacteria in your gut can and that may cause imbalances in your healthy gut flora.

What's more, it also causes oxidative stress and inflammation. Cancer cells feed upon sugar, especially fructose, and thrive in an oxidized environment.

Excess fructose also affects brain functioning, in terms of appetite regulation and blood sugar. In rats, it impairs memory.

I'm not trying to say that fruit is bar – just that excess fructose in the body comes with an array of negative side-effects and that it's not optimal for consumption. There are many people who eat a raw fruit based diet and seem to be perfectly fine. Comes to show that nutrition is highly individualized and even Keto Fasting may not suit everyone.

But still, on a fat burning metabolism, we can think more clearly and with less disruption. Our ability to concentrate increases and I dare say that so does our intelligence. Who knows, maybe our IQ gets raised by a few points so as well. Not directly, but as a result of being able to allocate our psychic energy into appropriate channels and activities that make us smarter. Personally, I've definitely noticed a lot of improvement in this area.

Sleep Like the Sleeping Beauty

Additionally, the quality of our sleep improves because of the stability in blood sugar. If we run out of glucose in the middle of the night, then we will become hypoglycemic. Our starving brain will wake us up to get some fuel. Midnight snacking is another example of people feeding all of the time and an extremely bad habit to have.

Constant stream of energy means that there's no need to recharge as much, resulting in quality slumber. This way we can go through full sleep cycles and actually enter the deepest stages of recovery where all dreaming occurs and the magic happens. During my own periods of ketosis, I've gone through the entire night like a log without waking up.

Sleep is one of the most important things for building muscle, getting stronger and burning fat. During the day we're exposing our body to all types of exhausting activities that push our limits to the extreme. Stress, exercise, thinking, traffic, mental algorithms, situational awareness, high digit numbers dinging all around us etc. are all draining us and not something we're supposed to be facing with on a daily basis. To actually cause enhanced physiological adaptations we have to allow the recovery processes to happen.

What you will also see is that you get less tired overall when on keto. Physical activities become less demanding and your endurance will increase by default. This is due to increased mitochondrial density, which is the topic of Chapter Eight. If you're obese, then you'll reclaim your enthusiasm and vitality for life. Being overweight means that you should be immediately put on a low carb diet. Physiologically, it doesn't make sense to keep fidgeting with insulin and sugar.

Once you go through the shift and eat appropriately, your body will heal itself. Inflammation disappears and you'll have less aches and pains. You may think that it's normal to be feeling the way you do now, but that's because you're unaware of another way.

All of these benefits are the reason why you should try a ketogenic diet... at least once. It will give you high end physical as well as cognitive performance and is incredibly healthy.

Being in this metabolic state is very advantageous, as we become more resourceful with our own supplies and can thus always be excelling at whatever we're doing. You're going to have to keep it a secret, but the military is also very interested of ketosis and is actively testing it on topnotch soldiers. When on keto, we literally can become Superhuman.

Chapter Takeaway

- Ketosis by default increases your fat oxidation and promotes fat loss.
- Ketogenic diets have been successfully used against diabetes, elevated blood glucose, cholesterol and

triglyceride levels, including many other cardiovascular diseases.

- When in ketosis, your body will have access to its infinite amount of stored calories and has more energy to use.
- Keto also promotes the healthy functioning of brain cells and has a positive effect on cognition.
- Fructose can only be metabolized by the liver and can't be converted into muscle glycogen. In excess, it can actually become toxic to the body.
- Nutritional ketosis maintains steady blood sugar and stable energy levels, thus allowing you to sleep better.

Chapter Four

Enter Fasting Fury

By now we've covered a whole lot but there's still more to learn. Keto is only one half to empowering our physiology and improving our performance. The other half is fasting, which we will go through in the following two chapters.

Contemporary medicine and the fitness industry have villainized fat but they have also stigmatized skipping meals. It's as if we are trying to eat all of the abundant food we're exposed to whereas we would be much better off by restricting our eating just a bit.

Re-Think Your Stance on Fasting (and Ketosis)

Before we go any further, it's important to dispel some of your pre-conceived notions about fasting and not eating. Maybe, in a not too distant past, you followed the Standard American Diet (SAD)[1], but have managed to drag yourself out from the jaws of death, literally. If you can accept keto, then it's much easier

---

[1] The SAD diet consists of refined carbohydrates, white sugar, white flour, processed meat, too much salt and dairy, with moderate amount of fruit and vegetables, low fat and protein.

to do the same with IF. Your immediate reaction might be: *"Who would be crazy enough to do this?"* It doesn't make any sense - at least that's what you might think. You need to wrap your head around fasting and change your idea about it. In contemporary nutrition circles it's 'the F word' - the forbidden fruit. *Don't skip a meal or else...*

The Difference Between Fasting and Starvation

We need to distinguish fasting from starvation. One is *voluntary* and *deliberate,* the other is *involuntary* and *forced upon.* It's like the difference between suicide and dying of old age.

Abstention from food is the art of manipulating our metabolic system and can be done for many reasons. Malpractice might look like the person is starving, but if done correctly it's very healthy and good for you.

Our body can only be in 2 metabolic states

- **Fasted** – meaning that there are no exogenous calories consumed at all.

- **Fed** – there are some calories circulating the blood stream.

Even consuming small amounts of food will put you into a fed state. <u>It doesn't matter whether you eat 200 calories or 1000, you'll still get kicked out of a fasted state.</u>

With that being said, you won't necessarily shift too far away from fasting physiology if you eat, let's say, 100 calories of 100% fat. If your blood sugar levels don't get elevated, then the calories consumed won't cross the blood-brain barrier either, making your brain think that no food was consumed. So there is a very narrow line between these two states and some room for maneuvering. More on this later.

Fasting is the Healthiest Way to Lose Weight

That's why intermittent fasting is a lot better than caloric restriction. If you're feeding yourself, but in inadequate amounts, then your body will most definitely perceive it as scarcity. You'll be causing more damage than good. If you do it the wrong way, you'll end up like someone from the concentration camps.

Daily caloric restriction decreases metabolism, so it's easy to presume that this would be magnified as food intake drops to zero. However, this is wrong. Once your food intake stops completely (you start to fast), the body shifts into ketosis. The hormonal adaptations of fasting will not occur by only lowering your caloric intake. In the case of being fasted, your physiology is under completely different conditions, which is unachievable by regular eating.

Starvation happens when there is not enough nutrition to be found *e.g.* when you go on a weight loss diet and restrict calories. While fasting, the organism is almost never deprived of essential nutrients, unless you lose all of your body fat. These fuel sources are mobilized from internal resources.

Fasting isn't a mechanism of starvation because your metabolism will be altered. This shift won't occur entirely if you continue consuming food, even when you've reduced your calories to a bare minimum. It's actually a lot healthier way of losing weight, as you'll be burning only fat, not muscle. When on a restrictive diet, you'll never make the leap and, to keep your energy demands at a balance, you begin to cannibalize your own tissue. When in a fasted state, this can be circumvented.

The Physiology of Fasting

Intermittent fasting (IF) is a way of eating (or not eating), where the food consumed is restricted to a certain time window. This means that no calories whatsoever get put into our body in any shape or form. In a way, it's simply timing when you eat. There are several patterns to this, all of which we will go through shortly.

The two governing states of metabolism are fed and fasted. The former is when we're using the macronutrients eaten, that have been digested and are now circulating the blood stream. The latter happens when all of that fuel has run out and our gas tank is empty, so to say. It happens after several hours (6-8) of not eating.

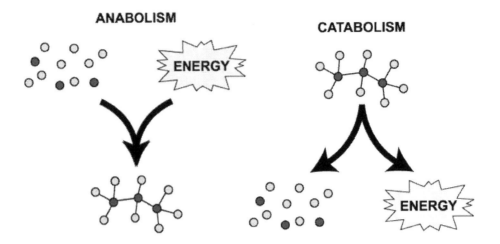

They're the different sides of the same coin. There are only two options: (1) eating and storing calories, (2) not eating and burning calories. Caloric restriction will still keep you in a fed state, a malnourished one, but still. Think of them as the Yin and Yang of metabolism.

You might think that no machine cannot operate without any energy. That's true only for mechanical things, but us humans are organic and a whole *'nother* being. Even though there is no fuel readily available, we're still able to function. In fact, to excel at it.

In a Fasted State There Are Several Ways to Produce Energy

The body's default fuel source is glucose, which exogenously (externally) comes in the form of sugar and carbohydrates and is stored endogenously as glycogen. The liver can deposit only 100-150 grams and our muscles about 300-500 grams. They're used for back-up.

Liver glycogen stores will be depleted already within the first 14 to 24 hours of not eating - almost overnight. This decreases blood sugar and insulin levels significantly, as there are no exogenous nutrients to be found.

Insulin is a hormone released by the pancreas in response to rising blood sugar, which happens after the consumption of food. Its role is to unlock the receptors in our cells to shuttle the incoming nutrients into our muscles, or when they're full into our adipose tissue (body fat).

The counterpart to insulin is glucagon and also gets produced by the pancreas. It gets released when the concentration of glucose in the blood stream gets too low. The liver then starts to convert stored glycogen into glucose.

This initial phase of fasting is characterized by a high rate of gluconeogenesis (the creation of new glucose) with the use of amino acids from bones and muscles.

Fasting and Ketosis

As fasting continues, the liver starts to produce ketone bodies which are derived from our own fat cells. Lipolysis and ketogenesis increase significantly due to fatty acid mobilization and oxidation.

Ketosis can occur already after 2-3 days of fasting. Triglycerides are broken down into glycerol, which is used for gluconeogenesis and broken down into three fatty acid chains. Fatty acids can be used for energy by most of the tissue in the body, but not the brain. They need to be converted into ketone bodies first.

Fasting induces ketosis very rapidly and puts the body into its more efficient metabolic state. Ketone bodies may rise up to 70-fold during prolonged fasting[xx].

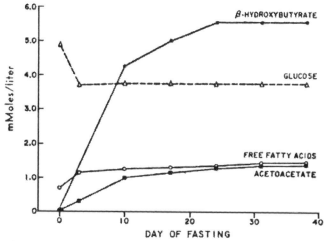

BLOOD GLUCOSE, FREE FATTY ACIDS
AND KETONE BODY LEVELS DURING FAST

FIG. 2. Circulating concentrations of βOHB, glucose, free fatty acids and acetoacetate in obese but otherwise normal man fasting for 40 days (9).

The more keto-adapted you become the more ketones you'll successfully utilize. At first, the brain and muscles are quite glucose dependent. But eventually they start to prefer fat for fuel.

After several days of fasting, approximately 75% of the energy used by the brain is provided by ketones. This also allows other species, such as king penguins, to survive for 5 months without any food[xxi].

Fasting also skyrockets human growth hormone exponentially within the first few days to maintain lean

body mass and muscle tissue. Afterwards it does so less significantly because protein catabolism gets reduced to almost non-existent levels. In this state, the majority of the body's energy demands will be met by the use of free fatty acids and ketones.

Why Fast

Now that we know what IF is, you might ask, why should we do it? Why abstain from eating voluntarily when it's readily available? That's a natural response.

Our species has followed the eating pattern of feast and famine ever since its genesis. Even today, hunter-gatherer societies have to fight for their food every single day and they sometimes can't make ends meet. They won't die because of that but instead simply get hungry from time to time.

In nature, food isn't as abundant as in our contemporary world of supermarkets. To be honest, it's an illusion, making us blind to how fortunate and unorthodox it actually is. Not only can we eat but also have a variety of products to choose from, too many, to be honest.

It's quite paradoxical that the majority of people in the world go to bed while starving every single night, but at the same time almost everyone in the Western society is obsessively obese.

The Pareto principle applies here perfectly[xxii]. He was an Italian economist and in his 1896 paper showed that, <u>in most cases, about 80% of the effects come from 20% of the causes</u>. 80% of the wealth belongs to 20% of the people, 80% of car accidents happen to 20% of the drivers, 80% of the food is consumed and stored as fat in 20% of the world's population etc. Mainly it's used in economics, but this 80-20 rule, or the law of the vital few, is evident in the distribution of calories and obesity as well.

Our civilization has reached a point where we don't have to worry about our most primary needs as much and can now spend more time on other activities that develop us further as a species – that is self-actualization. There's nothing wrong with that. In a perfect world, no animal would have to kill another one and everyone would always be fed and satisfied. However, we don't live in such a place yet, at least for the time being.

Nevertheless, despite the fact that we're surrounded by calories of all sort we still should do intermittent fasting. If you look at the rise in obesity and cardiovascular disease this abundance has bestowed us with then you definitely would realize the necessity of it for some people. However, these are only the obvious self-evident reasons. There are even more benefits to it which will improve the health and well-being of the lean individuals as well.

Chapter Takeaway

- Fasting isn't the same as starvation because your body will be under completely different metabolic conditions.
- You can either be in a fasted or fed state. Even eating just a little bit of calories will stop fasting and shifts your metabolism into digesting food.
- During fasting, your body can create energy from liver glycogen stores and ketone bodies.
- Fasting can induce ketosis already within 2-3 days. During that time, ketone bodies soar extremely high.
- Fasting also preserves lean muscle tissue due to the rise in growth hormone.

Chapter Five

The Effects of Fasting

Fasting completely alters the physiological conditions of our body. Most of it has to do with shifting into ketosis, which is achievable with a low carb diet as well. However, there are also other adaptations specifically characteristic to a purely fasted state.

The effects of fasting are very broad and cover both physical, mental and spiritual benefits. Once we stop eating for a while, our perspective on life changes and so does our body.

There are many beneficial and even empowering adaptations that occur during the abstinence from food. The most profound ones have to do with health, but they can also translate over to other domains as well.

Cellular Repair

Fasting is like a miracle cure, as many philosophers and physicians of the past would agree. The Renaissance doctor Paracelsus called it the *"physician within."* Because it triggers the body's own healing mechanisms it can be effectively used as treatment for almost any disease.

This is caused by the principle of '***autolysis,***' which is an organisms ability to selectively self-digest and remove unwanted material within the body, without touching vital structures.

When in a fasted state the body actually conducts a lot of the necessary repair mechanisms. It detoxifies the organism by triggering a metabolic pathway called '***autophagy,***' which removes waste material from cells[xxiii]. The word derives from Greek, meaning *auto (self) and phagein (to eat)* – literally "to eat oneself."

In autophagy, sub-cellular organelles are destroyed and new ones are built to replace them. Old cell membranes and other debris will then be removed. This happens through a specialized organelle called the '*lysosome,*' which contains enzymes that degrade proteins.

Increased levels of glucose, insulin and proteins all turn off autophagy. Even as little as 3 grams of the amino acid leucine can do so. When we eat carbs or protein, insulin gets released and a metabolic pathway called *'mammalian target of rapamycin'* (mTOR) gets activated. As a result, the body recognizes that there is food around and that decides to stop the removal of old cellular waste.

On the flip side, if mTOR is dormant and suppressed, autophagy gets promoted. In the absence of nutrients, the body needs to prioritize healthy organs and thus cycles out the worn out parts. They get transported to the liver where they will go through gluconeogenesis or get incorporated into new proteins. In the process, inflammation throughout the body and overall oxidative stress get reduced[xxiv]. This fights against all illnesses.

Disease is not a natural state to be in. The body is smart enough to fight it. We simply have to get out of our own way and let the automatic mechanisms set in to do their job. Constant eating directs all of our energy into digestion and doesn't create time for housekeeping. Because of the crap most people are eating, waste starts to accumulate and their body becomes a garbage bin. To prevent cancer and increase lifespan[xxv] we need to intermittently abstain from eating and recover[xxvi].

Increased Fat Oxidation

Fasting is also the healthiest and easiest way to reverse obesity. We already know about how bad caloric restriction is for us. <u>There's a big difference between losing weight and burning fat.</u> You probably know on which side you want to be.

You already know how fat storage and mobilization works but it doesn't harm us to re-iterate it once again. Before you can burn fat, you have to first "release" the fatty acids into your blood stream through via lipolysis. They then get transported to the mitochondria where they'll be oxidized into energy. Another essential component to this is hormone-sensitive lipase, which permits the mobilization of body fat. If insulin and blood glucose levels are high, even in a caloric deficit, then this will be completely inhibited and mobilizing fat out of the adipocytes will become essentially impossible for several days to come. That is why I'm a big proponent of low carb ketogenic diets as well because they put your body into its *prime-primal* metabolic state – that's what Keto Fasting does.

During rest, our muscles start to use more fatty acids for fuel. When fat burning increases so does the amount of Uncoupling Protein-3 in our muscles. As little as 15-hours of fasting enhances the gene expression for UP-3 by 5-fold[xxvii]. It's function is to protect the mitochondria from stress. We'll be using ketones to feed our lean tissue more effectively.

In a fasted state we begin to use our own body fat as fuel. This not only promotes body composition but also teaches us to produce energy despite the lack of calories. As a result, we experience less hunger and fatigue by not being dependent of food in order to feel great. It's an important and vital thing for our survival, which we don't want to lose.

By being constantly fed, we're never really converting fatty acids into the blood stream and are simply burning the food we've digested. This will definitely slow down weight loss, if not put a harsh halt to it completely. In the case of an unexpected famine we would be dumbstruck for a while because our body doesn't have enough reference experience. <u>In a nutshell – fasting allows your body to take a break from storing fat, and start burning it.</u>

Hastened Metabolism

Contrary to popular belief, intermittent fasting doesn't slow down the metabolism but actually increases it by 3.6% after the first 48 hours[xxviii]. Even further, 4 days in, resting energy expenditure increases up to 14%[xxix].

Instead of slowing down the metabolism, the body revs it up and puts it into higher gear. This is probably caused by increased adrenaline so that we would have more energy to go out into the savannah and find some food. The scarcer calories become the more detrimental it is to succeed in hunting.

People think that if they skip breakfast the body will hold onto its own body fat and store every calorie in the next meal. Think about it. Does your body really think it's starving after not eating for a day or is it simply your primal mind playing tricks on you? Like said, the pattern of feast and famine is something our species is adapted to. It's just that people have lost these pathways of fat oxidation and think they're dying when they don't eat 6 meals a day. Their metabolism simply needs to be made more resilient.

Reduced Cholesterol

How Does Fasting Reduce Cholesterol?

Most of the body's cholesterol gets created by the liver, thus eating less cholesterol has almost no effect on its production. In fact, it may be actually counter-productive. As the liver senses less incoming cholesterol, it may rev up its own production, leading to health problems and the clogging of arteries.

During fasting, you're not consuming any dietary carbohydrates and the liver will thus decrease its synthesis of triglycerides. Excess carbohydrates that cannot be stored within the body will be converted into triglycerides. Therefore, the absence of carbohydrates means fewer triglycerides. Triglycerides are released from the liver as *'very low density lipoproteins'* (VLDLs), which are a precursor for the formation of *'low density lipoproteins'* (LDL - "bad" cholesterol). On top of that, fasting preserves *'high density lipoproteins'* (HDL - "good" cholesterol).

Fights Diabetes

In type-1 diabetes the body's own immune system destroys the insulin producing cells in the pancreas. The resulting low insulin levels lead to high blood sugar. Therefore, since insulin levels are low to begin with, you would want to use supplemental insulin to reduce blood sugar.

In type-2 diabetes, insulin levels are not low but high. Blood sugar is elevated not because the body can't make insulin but because it's become resistant to insulin. In this case, elevating insulin makes matters only worse. Insulin causes insulin resistance and the safest way to treat diabetes is to keep blood sugars low without tampering with insulin.

Increased Insulin Sensitivity

In a fasted state, we actually become more efficient with the food we eat, instead of storing it all. With the lack of calories, especially carbohydrates, we become more insulin sensitivity[xxx], meaning that we need less of it to lower our blood sugar levels back to normal. In the case of resistance, the pancreas can't pump out enough to get the job done, which leads to hypertension and disease. Fasting can actually reverse insulin resistance and reduces overall blood sugar levels.

Lowering insulin gets rid of excess salt and water in the body, which is caused by carbohydrates in the first place. Insulin is the key hormone in the regulation of our metabolism and the main driver of obesity and diabetes. Fasting and a low carb diet are great ways of controlling its expression.

There's no reason to be concerned about malnutrition during fasting, because our fat stores can deposit almost an infinite amount of calories. The main issue is rather micronutrient deficiencies.

Potassium levels may drop slightly, but even 2 months of fasting don't decrease it below a safe margin. Magnesium, calcium and phosphorus remain stable because 99% of them are stored in our bones. The longest recorded fast lasted for 382 days and was maintained, with no harmful effects on the subject's health, thanks to taking a simple multivitamin[xxxi]. That's all you need to survive for that long.

Boosts Human Growth Hormone

Another anabolic mechanism that gets increased is human growth hormone (HGH). <u>After 14-18 hours of fasting it does so by an astonishing 1300-2000%</u>[xxxii]. It not only promotes tissue repair, body composition and metabolism but also preserves youthfulness. The hormone of eternal youth – the Holy Grail Hormone of longevity.

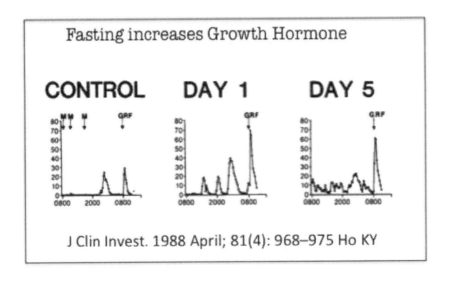

J Clin Invest. 1988 April; 81(4): 968–975 Ho KY

Growth hormone plays a key role in the metabolism of all macronutrients. Its normal secretion fluctuates throughout the day and increases significantly during the first hours of sleep at about 11-12 PM.

After 3 days of fasting, HGH increases dramatically in non-obese individuals, but flats out after day 10[xxxiii][xxxiv]. In obese people, there is little to no reported rise after fasting from 14 to 38 days [xxxv]. Hypothetically, this happens as a response to preserving lean tissue. I would suggest that beyond that point the body simply becomes extremely well keto adapted and reduces both the overall energy demands as well as increases the efficient use of ketones as fuel, so there is little to no need for that much growth hormone.

Exogenous growth hormone supplementation and injections have an array of unwanted consequences, such as an increase in blood sugar levels, higher blood pressure, risk of prostate cancer and heart problems.

Eating suppresses the secretion of growth hormone and so does overeating. The best natural way to stimulate growth hormone is to do fasting. Funny enough, low calorie diets don't cause the same response - because you're either fed or fasted.

IGF-1

What goes hand in hand with HGH is insulin-like growth factor (IGF-1). It's one of the major growth factors in mammals, which together with insulin, is associated with accelerated aging and cancer. Just 5 days of fasting can decrease it by 60% and cause a 5-fold increase one of its principal IGF-1-inhibiting proteins: IGFBP1[xxxvi].

By the same token, it's an all-encompassing anabolic hormone, like insulin, that makes everything within the body grow – the good (muscle), the bad (fat cells) and the ugly (tumors). It gets reduced during fasting but also gets stimulated by it, as with physical training.

Additionally, testosterone increases as well. During my 48-hour fasts I usually experience higher libido than normally. Even though there's no direct reason for it, I have a feeling of risen masculinity and T-levels. It's not aggressive energy, but more like my determination heightens and focus narrows down completely.

Intermittent fasting creates the perfect environment for anabolism not catabolism as a lot of people think. Being constantly fed results in the over-expression of insulin and IGF-1, which is not optimal for overall health. You want to activate these powerful steroid hormones in very specific conditions. Occasional fasting is a great way to control and use them only when you want to.

You don't have to take supplemental steroids to release these anabolic hormones. They're already a part of our physiology. We simply have to turn on some of our genetic switches and become fat burning beasts.

Longevity and Life-Span

Fasting induces oxidative stress because of producing a surge in free radicals - the molecules mostly associated with aging. This further stimulates a gene called SIRT3[xxxvii] to increase the production of 'sirtuins,' which are protective proteins of longevity. In mice they extend lifespan. There are no studies in humans but the effects may be similar.

The rise in free radicals is actually beneficial because they trigger protective pathways. If the body is intermittently exposed to low levels of oxidative stress it can build a better response and cope with it better.

When you abstain an organism from calories for a certain period of time, their expected life span will increase by 30%, but they will eventually still starve to death.

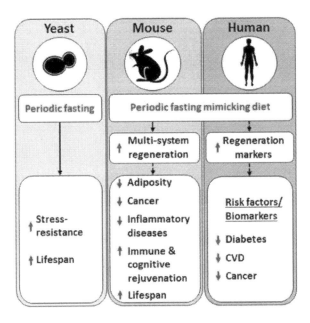

The key to actually gaining any benefits from this abstinence is to do it intermittently – that is to practice fasting and feasting. Eating one meal a day is also a great way to take advantage of both these mechanisms, namely improved longevity and sustenance.

Extended life span is the biggest reason why I think intermittent fasting is so important. Think about it, you can potentially live a whole lot longer by simply abstaining from eating every now and then. What's more, your overall existential experience will actually improve.

On top of that, autophagy and insulin sensitivity keep the body clean and healthy. Too much junk will damage our mitochondria – the power plants of our cells. Ketosis actually increases our mitochondrial density, giving us more energy, and so does intermittent fasting. The combination of those two can help us live a lot longer whilst being able to maintain our vigor.

Having combined both of these strategies I definitely feel like I've put a halt to my aging process almost entirely, at least slowed it down significantly. I'm still 22 and I shouldn't show any signs of getting older in the first place, but based on my gut feeling I'm expecting to live past 150.

My insulin is never elevated for the majority of the time and my blood is clean of free radicals. After ditching the carbs, eating a lot of healthy fats and doing intermittent fasting, my skin has never been clearer and my nails are perfect.

Rejuvenescence

By the same token, fasting has a characteristic that's perfectly natural to life. It's the ability of living things to regain youthfulness. This physiological term is called 'rejuvenescence.'

Experimental scientists have demonstrated this on lower forms of life. They deprive some creatures back from adulthood to their embryonic stages of life, as if they were reborn. This has been done several times, meaning that the animal has reached an old age and then been reverted back to its youth, over and over again. That's quite amazing.

For humans this probably won't work... yet... but man can definitely benefit from the same physiological characteristics. At the University of Chicago, Carlson and Kunde fasted a 40-

year old male for two weeks and discovered that his cellular physiology was that of a 17-year old. This happens by ridding the cells of toxic metabolic accumulates that impede your bioenergetics.

One of the features of youthfulness is seen in the cell to nucleus ratio. Youthful cells have a preponderance of nuclear material, while old and senile cells have a dominance of cellular material. Autophagy keeps the cells refreshed and circulates between old and new building blocks.

Fasting will also rejuvenate your psychological youthfulness. You get a breath of fresh air and can give your brain some reasons to enhance its functioning. Frequent eating also dulls the mind and makes you mentally more slothful. The hungry hunter's cognition was as sharp as a knife.

Cancer and Tumors

There are some good reasons to consider fasting as something that could potentially cure cancer or definitely alleviate its symptoms. One of the first studies in this field showed that it not only prolonged life but reduced the prevalence of breast cancer tumors in rats[xxxviii]. Another one done on mice found out that 48-hour fasting effectively protected normal cells but not cancer cells against high doses of chemotherapy and also alleviated its side-effects.

The reason might be that there's simply not enough food for cancer cells to feed upon. While fasting, blood glucose levels drop and ketone concentration increases. The #1 fuel for tumors is sugar and they commit cellular suicide through starvation. It probably isn't enough to cure the disease completely in humans, but it's a step in the right direction.

For healthy people, intermittent fasting can instead be used as disease prevention. Increased insulin sensitivity and *autophagy* are quite good predictors of longevity. It's the most natural antioxidant there is. It heals, repairs and regenerates the body. These qualities are greatly enhanced during a fast and can cure diseases that don't go away while eating.

Dominic D'Agostino is one of the leading researchers in the field of nutritional ketosis and cancer treatment. He practices keto himself and also does a lot of intermittent fasting. His advice for everyone is to do therapeutic fasting 1-3 times per year to purge precancerous cells and reboot the immune system. The fasts should last for 3-5 days because autophagy starts to really ramp up only after the first 24 hours. Chapter Five in Part Two gives you the 2 Day Fast Formula.

Bolstered Brain Power

While intermittent fasting, we will experience mental clarity. It also increases levels of a hormone called *'brain-derived neurotrophic factor'* (BDNF)[xxxix], a deficiency of which has been implicated in depression and various other similar problems.

New brain neurons get formulated, which is a process called *'neurogenesis'* Intermittent fasting makes one mentally sharp and reduces brain fog. It sharpens cognition, increases learning memory and enhances synaptic plasticity[xl], improves our stress tolerance[xli] and protects against neurodegenerative disease[xlii]. Ketosis may increase seizure thresholds in epileptic patients as well, which is stimulated by fasting.

Evolutionarily it promoted ingenuity – to find new ways to getting food, making better traps, come up with more lethal hunting strategies etc. When faced with famine, the only way to survive was to get smarter.

Fasting can be used as a way to boost your mental powers. Artists and writers in the past usually abstained from eating during their most creative circuits. Michelangelo painted the ceiling of the Sistine Chapel vigorously day and night, rarely coming down to eat or even sleep. Pythagoras the Ancient Greek mathematician routinely fasted for 40 days in a row, saying that it allowed him to remain mentally sharp. All of the other philosophers, such as Socrates and Plato also preached fasting for greater cognitive clarity.

After the body has shifted from using glucose to burning fat for fuel, appetite gets reduced dramatically. This is because the brain gets abundant energy from ketones. You'll be able to direct your psychic energy onto other more demanding activities.

What follows is a sense of well-being and euphoria. The explanation might be that the accumulation of acetoacetic acid produces a mild intoxication similar to that of ethanol[xliii]. You'll be literally high on keto.

Advantages of Fasting

In addition to all of the physiological benefits mentioned already, fasting has a ton of advantages on all aspects of your life.

- **Fasting is extremely effective and simple**. It doesn't take a rocket scientist to practice IF because all you have to do is... not eat. A full on caloric ban during certain eating windows is actually a lot more liberating than having to eat several times per day. That's why so many people can't ever seem to stick to their diet or lose weight – they're simply overwhelmed by counting calories and timing their meals.
- **IT'S FREE.** You don't need to pay anyone to cook your meals or spend money on buying a ton of groceries every single day. It's the cheapest way of losing weight and improving your health. Burn calories not cash. #tweet that @inthevanguard

- **You save a lot of time**. By the same token, you don't have to waste a lot of valuable time on meal prepping, cooking three course dinners or eating, for a fact. It's super convenient to skip a meal whenever you don't feel like having one. My greatest productivity hack is <u>my one meal a day</u>. I don't eat breakfast because it would rob me precious hours in the morning, during which I do most of my creative work. For me, food slows me down – IF and keto allow me to keep my killer instinct alive.

- **Enjoy an occasional splurge and indulgence**. Dieting doesn't mean you have to necessarily give up your favourite foods. Thanks to the medicinal benefits of fasting, you can easily have your cake and eat it too while still getting away with it. Fasting is a great addition to any diet program. However, you won't be able to maintain ketosis if you go about eating everything in sight. It's just that you can structure it into your strategy and not suffer any severe consequences. What's best though is that, once you keto-adapt you'll lose the desire to cheat all together and wouldn't want to trade a short sugar rush for the amazing satiety you feel on keto.

Potential Side-Effects

There may, however, be some negative consequences to fasting. Headaches, dizziness, lightheadedness, fatigue, low blood pressure and abnormal heart rhythms are all short-term. Some people may experience impaired motor control or forgetfulness.

But these are all symptoms of withdrawal, not fasting. Because most people rarely get to use their own body fat for fuel, they become too dependent of glucose. It's like an addiction that makes them crave more sugar.

When I first started practicing intermittent fasting I experienced some hypoglycemia (low blood sugar response) but nothing serious. I simply got a bit lightheaded whenever I stood up too fast. After going on a ketogenic diet, those signs have disappeared completely.

Any mental hindrance is caused by an inner energy crisis. Once the body adapts to utilizing fat for fuel, the brain will accept ketones and also reduces hunger. It creates this omni-focused and self-motivated state of mind, during which you won't get distracted by food and can concentrate on whatever you want.

Fasting may cause flare-ups of certain medical conditions, such as gout, gallstones or other diseases. This is yet again not because of the physiological effect of fasting but because of the overall high amounts of toxins in the body. The adipose tissue is more than a caloric pantry. It also stores poisons and infections that we digest. The food we eat is the most immediate point of contact we have with the world around us. Unlike the skin, our gut is the one that absorbs all of the molecules. Once you start breaking down triglycerides from your adipose tissue, those same toxins will be released into your blood stream again and need to get flushed out. There may also be some nervous stomach, irritable bowel or diarrhea. That's why fasting is an effective detox tool, as it cleanses the organism completely.

Another negative side-effect of fasting is the feeling of being more cold. This may be catalyzed by several reasons but the main cause is reduced metabolic rate. If our metabolism slows down, we will start to shiver, get tired, hungry and less energetic - our body is trying to conserve energy by not burning calories to keep us warm and moving. This happens not due to the intrinsic effects of fasting but because of the state of an organism's own inner physiology. <u>If your hormones are *out of whack* and you have very little body fat, then your body will compensate by making you feel colder.</u> To alleviate that you would want to dial down on your overall cortisol and limit your fasting because it's still a stressor like any other.

Essential nutrients, especially nitrogen can be lost through urine during fasting. Nitrogen in the urine is a sign of protein metabolism, and as protein metabolism decreases during fasting, nitrogen excretion decreases significantly as well. To not lose too many micronutrients or become mineral deficient you can supplement with a multivitamin that doesn't have calories or spike your insulin (more on supplementation in Chapter Seven of Part Three), or drink a cup of homemade bone broth daily (Chapter Six).

In comparison to all of the empowering health benefits of fasting, these few side-effects are minute and not guaranteed.

They may or may not happen. What's certain is that they will be alleviated after time.

Why then have we been lead to believe that fasting is bad for us? Medical doctors and supplement companies all preach the consumption of 6 small meals a day. Why? I'm not going to be pointing any fingers or calling anyone out, but simply put: there's no money to be made from healthy people. How do you prescribe a pill of fasting that's completely free?

Fasting is perfectly natural and incredibly powerful tool for many purposes. The most obvious ones have to do with body composition and fat reduction. For someone like me who is already as lean as I can be, the best benefits have to do with using ketones as fuel and increased longevity. It's one of the staples in my nutritional arsenal and something we should all be doing, no matter our condition.

Chapter Takeaway

- Fasting induces cellular repair and detox via autophagy. This will purge precancerous cells and resets the immune system.

- Your metabolic rate doesn't decrease but actually increases after fasting for 48-hours.
- Growth hormone increases by 1300-2000% during fasting and is the perfect way to promote building lean muscle, burning fat and increasing longevity.
- Fasting fights against many diseases, such as diabetes, increased cholesterol and insulin resistance.
- Abstention from food will increase your life span and boosts youthfulness.
- Fasting can also bolster your brain against neurodegenerative disease and will sharpen your focus.
- The potential side-effects of fasting are mostly withdrawal symptoms from burning glucose and consequences of having an unhealthy body in the first place.

Chapter Six

The Breakfast Myth

"It's the most important meal of the day! Wake up, eat a lot of fruit and cereal to kickstart your metabolism and give yourself energy!" You've probably heard this from nutritionists and fitness gurus countless times. To be honest, I'm quite sick of it.

Actually, they're right. Breakfast is indeed the most important meal of the day, as it determines our metabolic state for the rest of the day, as well as the next. However, it doesn't mean we should be having it.

Eating first thing in the morning doesn't have any beneficial effects. After an overnight's fast, we're in an advantageous state of increased fat oxidation. Our liver glycogen stores have been depleted and we're in mild ketosis.

Within a few hours, other hormonal activities will speed up and we'll empower our body. Growth hormone gets released and our insulin sensitivity improves. Also, testosterone increases and our cells go through the repair mechanisms of autophagy. The reason is that the body is in a semi-catabolic state and will become more efficient with nutrient partitioning and shifts into a higher gear of fat burning.

Having breakfast with a lot of sugary cereal, fruit, or a whole grain bagel will put a harsh stop to all of these adaptations. Tony the Tiger is wrong - *It's not grrrreat!* Causing an insulin response at any other time of the day can prevent fat burning completely or at least slow it down significantly. Another reason why you would want to eat a ketogenic diet.

The stress hormone cortisol is also the highest. It rises at about 6-8 AM so that we could become more alert for the coming day. This increases our adrenaline and fat oxidation even further. Why not take advantage of this short boost? It would be a shame to pass out on all of these adaptations. The stage is set - we just have to get out of our own way.

When you go to bed at night, you release the most growth hormone. Having fasted in the morning, you condition your body to do it more than 1300-2000%[xliv]. If you ate, then you won't be doing it nearly as much.

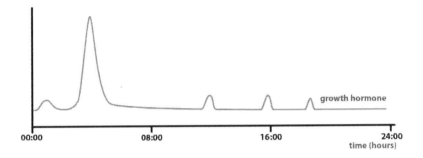

00:00   08:00   16:00   24:00
                                              time (hours)

Hunger Is a Circadian Signal

There is also a circadian rhythm to hunger (day and night cycles), with a ditch at 8AM and a peak at 8PM[xlv]. A study found that despite the extended overnight fast, paradoxically, people aren't as ravenous in the morning and they tend to not want much breakfast. You'd think that the longer they've spent fasting the hungrier they'd get, but the opposite happened. No matter how long their fast had lasted, the participants still reported less desire to eat after waking up. Instead, the internal clock increased appetite in the evening, independent of food intake and other factors. This makes perfect sense, as after an overnight fast we're in mild ketosis and utilizing fat for fuel. It also means that no matter how much whole grain cereal you stuff down your throat once you open your eyes, you'll still get hungry by the evening. The difference is that you'll have skipped all of the hormonal adaptations and have already consumed a lot of calories during the day.

This I've noticed in my own hunger signaling as well. In the morning, I don't have a lot of desire to eat immediately. Only after taking the first mouthful does the desire arise. Before that, I'm actually very satisfied and don't even notice any difference. It probably has to do with the fact that we've been conditioned by our society to start feeding right away. The work horse has to be just nourished enough to do its job. If it gets too strong and powerful though it may become a problem...

Why is it thought that you would gain weight if you eat in the evening? It's probably based on past experiences. But that knowledge has nothing to do with meal timing. Instead, people gain weight when they have big dinners because they've already spent the majority of the day feasting. Having breakfast, lunch and multiple snacks in between will have already made them consume a lot of calories. Now, they've already reached their caloric maintenance and can easily go over to a surplus. They simply don't have a nutritional plan and are randomly winging it.

That's why I would always recommend not having breakfast. In reality, we can never really skip it as the first thing we put into our mouths, despite the time, will shift our metabolism from being fasted into a fed state. We're simply having it later in the day and still getting our nutrients.

Why Am I Hungry?

Hunger is created by the hormone called ghrelin, that is produced by the gut to stimulate appetite. It signals the brain that the body is running low on fuel and it is time to eat something.

However, it doesn't necessarily mean that there is an energy crisis. It's more like a pre-cautionary message that lets us know when we have reached the lower ends of our immediately accessible fuel tank. Think of it like the gas light of your car.

The biggest reason why us humans have to eat so many calories is to feed our hungry brain. It's the most expensive tissue we have. Making up less than 5% of our body weight, it demands about 20% of our total energy expenditure.

Leptin resistance and the release of ghrelin happen because of the brain perceiving energy as scarcity. These hormones ought to motivate us to consume more food, even when there's no immediate necessity for it. We'll happily store any excess into our adipose tissue.

However, the brain shouldn't require a lot of calories to maintain its functioning. Once our immediate access to energy within the body has run out, we still have a lot of stored fuel with us.

From the perspective of evolution, we shouldn't experience hunger because of facing exhaustion. The energy stored in our adipose tissue would keep us alive but we still get hungry. Looking at how large our fuel tank really is, it seems that the issue isn't how many calories we have but how effectively we use them.

If you think that you have to eat first thing in the morning, then riddle me this: *"Why do you think you need to have breakfast?"*

The reason can't be to prevent yourself from starving to death. Nor can it be to *"kickstart your metabolism"* or prevent gaining fat. When you look at my body composition, which is at single digits year-round, and how much I train, which is every day, then the reason can't have anything to do with some sort of an advantageous metabolic state.

My body is constantly under very demanding conditions, yet I do not suffer any negative effects of undereating. I'm incredibly lean, muscular, strong and fit – all while not having breakfast. Please, tell me more that you need to stop your muscles from cannibalizing themselves and prevent yourself from getting fat.

The reason why you think that you may break down your own muscle is that your body doesn't know how to use its own stored fuel. Our adipose tissue can deposit almost an infinite amount of energy. Even the leanest of individuals with less than 7% body fat carry around more than 20 000 calories with them at all times. What about those who are overweight then?

Experiments of prolonged fasting on obese people show that they get hungry once their adipose tissue gets depleted and they reach lower amounts of body fat. This happens in conjunction with increased Neuropeptide Y. In the Bible, Jesus was said to have fasted for 40 days and 40 nights, before he got hungry.

You get hungry because you can't access your infinite supply source of energy. This is the result of contemporary eating habits, such as snacking and having 6 small meals a day. Frequent eating will never lead to complete satiety. Even when you have one big meal at lunch, you will still continue to crave food because you're used to having it very often. Remember, the body adapts to exactly the conditions it gets exposed to.

Let's think very deeply about hunger for a moment. What does it feel like? It's a sensation you get in your stomach - a surge of ghrelin that makes you growl and motivated to eat. But there's a huge BUT here. <u>The way you experience hunger is always the same from a physical perspective - whether that be while fasting or eating several times a day.</u> The signals are the same in both cases. The difference is only a matter of degree. When you haven't eaten anything for 5 hours, then you get the same sensation when you would have been fasting for several days. What we think is hunger is not actually hunger.

What Causes Sugar Cravings

The same thing applies to sugar cravings. Every time we consume something sweet, the reward endorphins in our brain light up.

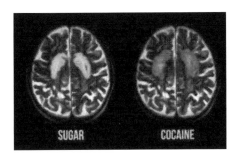

Remember this? In neurological terms, binge eating and drug addiction are the same thing[xlvi].

This happens so that we would be motivated to repeat our actions in the future. Our taste buds are designed to recognize sweetness and fire up every single time. Feeling good after eating something sugary puts us on a short high and makes us want more.

At the same time, that quick burst of energy will meet its quick downfall. After eating carbohydrates, our blood sugar levels rise. In response, the pancreas releases insulin to lower it back to normal. As a result, we will experience a drop, because insulin is clearing our blood stream from glucose and shuttling it into either muscle or fat cells.

This sharp high is followed by a steep low that causes mild hypoglycemia - a drop in blood sugar levels that makes us feel sleepy and drowsy instead of energized.

Now the body is facing an energy crisis. The brain will then scream out for more energy. Because the best fuel source it can think of is glucose, it will create sugar cravings.

The reason for sugar cravings is to make the body search for easily storable energy and to prevent hypoglycemia.

However, both of them are not justifiable in most situations. If a person has a lot of body fat, then they are carrying around stored energy with them at all times. Yet they can't seem to lose sugar cravings at night. Any other time of the day, really.

Sugar cravings are an effective evolutionarily stable strategy, but only in environments where finding energy is difficult. Calories in the modern world are more than abundant.

You shouldn't have sugar cravings or feel hungry after a meal at all because of just having consumed calories. If you do, then you might have some blood sugar problems.

To get rid of sugar cravings and reduce the feeling of hunger, we have to teach our body to burn fat instead. Becoming *'fat-adapted'* means that we know how to use fat for fuel very efficiently. As a result, we will have access to almost an infinite amount of calories stored in our adipose tissue.

Intermittent fasting is a great strategy for reversing leptin resistance and reducing the expression of ghrelin. If you want to completely free yourself from sugar addiction, then **you need to reset your body's taste buds.**

Following a short period of ketogenic eating acts like a sugar detox. You'll clear your liver and muscle cells from excess glucose and begin to use fat as fuel. This will truly liberate your mind as well from wanting carbohydrates and makes your body independent of sugar.

Your bliss point gets lowered, but your happiness will increase. Imagine how good you'll feel once you get out of the rut of craving more and more stimulation without ever reaching satisfaction. Ridding yourself from the desire is where the solution lies. Go straight to the root problem, which is inefficient energy usage, and don't simply alleviate the symptoms.

These metabolic pathways don't happen in of themselves and need to be tapped into. You have to teach your body how to burn fat and a period of adaptation is necessary. That's why you should do the ketogenic diet at least once, as it will reset your body and reinvigorates your fat burning mechanisms.

Is Skipping Breakfast Bad

It's true that your basal metabolic rate may slightly decrease with less frequent eating. But that's not necessarily a bad thing nor will it equal fat gain. The question we should all be asking isn't: *"How many calories I can potentially consume while not gaining fat?"* but: *"How less calories can I get away with while not losing lean muscle or damaging my health?"*

You begin to need fewer calories not because your body is starving but because your metabolism gets more effective. Occasional intermittent fasting will initially speed up the process by 3-14%. A kickstart is needed only when there's a necessity for it. Small meals will allow your body to become slothful, whereas it's better to be sharp and poised for immediate action. With enough conditioning you'll be able to plug into the largest fuel tank of them all.

However, skipping breakfast doesn't work for everyone due to their medical condition or lifestyle. The purpose of this chapter isn't to stigmatize eating in the morning. Instead, it's a call to action to start restricting your feeding window and to practice intermittent fasting. You shouldn't eat throughout the day if you want to do Keto Fasting.

The desire to have breakfast is therefore not caused by physiological necessity but by psychological hunger.

These two things are distinct from one another. They also include the notions of self-mastery and higher levels of consciousness.

Physiological Hunger	Psychological Hunger
• Empty feeling in the stomach • Stomach pangs • Light headedness • Headache or irritability	• You are not physiologically hungry • If you wait, the hunger goes away • Is emotionally triggered through sight, smell, or habit

Most people eat simply out of boredom. They have nothing else to do other than to walk between the fridge and the couch. This is sad and should be addressed immediately. Snacking is already one of the worst habits to have. It has nothing to do with needing energy. If you feel like it, then you should practice intermittent fasting. This goes straight to the underlying issue, which is your body's inability to use its own fat for fuel.

Are You Afraid of Hunger?

This almost phobic fear of going hungry is completely irrational. Our society is already teaching us that we should eat frequently and an empty stomach is a dangerous sign of starvation. In reality, it activates our primal instinct and puts us into hunger mode, in which we're more alert, stronger and sharper. Fasting makes us *hungrier for life*. (#tweet that

@inthevanguard) If you're controlled by it and give in too easily, then you're being enslaved by your urges.

First, you should realize that it's not going to harm you. It's mainly a brief sensation that occurs according to your habitual eating schedule. Your body is simply asking you, whether or not you still remember that previously it has received food at this exact moment. If you skip this urge, then you're conditioning yourself to not be influenced by it.

Fasting allows you to re-conceptualize hunger. Instead of linking it with panic, lethargy and desire[xlvii], it can be associated with success, self-mastery, pride, or simply ignored. You'll actually become more mindful of your urges and realize that most of the time you're following your habitual eating patterns.

Have the right mindset - be mentally as well as physically prepared to handle the hunger. Rather than being scared of it, you have to re-conceptualize it in your own head. Society has led us to think that a growling empty stomach is a sign of starvation with detrimental consequences to your health. In reality, it's anything but that, if it's done correctly and if you're in control of your environment.

Excruciating hunger with pain involved is a different story. It probably won't happen during fasting, but only when your body is chronically depleted of essential nutrients. Self-mastery is about controlling not torturing yourself. You should listen to your urges and understand them correctly. Learn how to differentiate between physiological hunger and psychological cravings.

Be More Mindful, Be More Human

I despise mindless eating on the run as well. Simply putting something into your mouth doesn't mean that your mind actually realizes that you've been fed. The scavenger is the one who has to take an advantage of every opportunity of eating in sight. It can't realize that food doesn't equal scarcity and that skipping a meal isn't bad. The predator knows that going hungry will only strengthen its instinct and won't gorge itself.

A Short Mind-Trip

Imagine yourself being obese and watching TV. Next to you is a bag of chips, which you're constantly digging into. One handful after another you keep on shoveling that food into your throat without even noticing it. At one point you reach the bottom and open up another bag – the vicious cycle continues. As sad as it seems, there are too many people like this. They already have leptin resistance and it's only a matter of time until diabetes and other cardiovascular diseases catch up with them.

I would much rather make every meal special and savor it. Rather than eating mindlessly, we should bring our complete attention to the dish. Follow along with me on yet another short fantasy mind-trip. Smell the aroma of your favorite food. Is it steaming hot, or something cold? Allow your taste buds to already light up before you even take a bite. The juices are flowing in your mouth and you look at the plate in front of you. It's a beautiful sight, especially if you're breaking your fast. You're already anticipating your first mouthful but don't get too attached to it. Let your motive be in the act itself, not the reward.

As Leonardo da Vinci said: *"The average person looks without seeing, listens without hearing, touches without feeling, eats without tasting, moves without physical awareness, inhales without awareness of odour or fragrance, and talks without thinking."*

In addition to mindless eating, we're being less mindful in all areas of our life. People don't know how to control their emotions because of having distanced themselves from their physiology. Fasting re-creates this intimate relationship we all should have with our body.

Mindfulness is about being aware of oneself in the present. It's recognizing what goes on in our immediate surroundings and being capable of creating modules of ourselves in the future to come. In so doing, you're raising your level of consciousness, which is the creation of your higher self, the pre-frontal cortex and even beyond that.

As you're reading these lines, are you completely present? Can you truly say that you're entirely HERE and in the NOW.

Take a notice of what goes on around you. What are the sounds you hear in your ears, the smells you smell with your nose like?

Bring your total attention to the soles of your feet, your breath and be aware.

More importantly, what goes on inside you? What sort of feelings and sensations are you having? Are you being controlled by your moods, or have you managed to achieve self-mastery and rise above them?

Rather than falling victim to our ego and getting high-jacked by our emotions, we have to opportunity to take control of them. Mindfulness enables us to always behave from the perspective of our higher self. It's what makes us human.

Eat your food and be grateful for it. Feel how the flavors enroll in your mouth – salty, sour, tenderness, not too much and not too little. Before going for another mouthful, enjoy the moment and let the current stimulus to pass (it takes about 10-15 seconds). You don't have to do this in slow motion, as it might look like in your head. Eat at normal speed, but at the same time be completely mindful of the process.

For me, skipping breakfast is incredibly enjoyable and easy. During my morning hours I get the most of my creative work done. In fact, it's 9AM as I'm writing this book. My mind is extra sharp and I'm able to formulate top notch literature, *sans food*. Leonardo himself practiced fasting and he was a genius.

Think how much more productive we can be by eating less often. Food is like a civilization's obsession. Don't get me wrong again. I love eating as well as cooking. On top of being a writer I also consider myself an up to par chef. It's almost therapeutic and a special occasion. But it's just that – a significant event that picks up its value only because of its low frequency. If I were to do it 3 times a day I wouldn't enjoy it nearly as much.

With intermittent fasting you don't have to think about meal prepping either. I've never been one of those guys who cooks all of their meals of the week and packs them into Tupperware. Who would want to eat that? Of course you can heat it up but when you're on the run you would have to consume it cold. That's not very tasty. A scavenger eats carcasses that have been left to rot. The predator eats a fresh kill with the blood being still warm.

Ultimately, you have to come to terms with what relationship you want to have with food. Do you eat to live or live to eat?

Intermittent fasting can improve your health, body composition and eating habits. At the same time, it enables you to still enjoy delicious meals. Actually, the quality and taste of them gets better. As the saying goes: *"You never know what a good meal tastes like, until you haven't had it for a long time."*

Chapter Takeaway

- Eating breakfast first thing in the morning doesn't have any metabolic advantage. In fact, you'll be skipping out on a lot of the hormonal adaptations that occur with fasting.
- Hunger is a circadian signal that gets released by our habitual way of eating.
- We get hungry not because of facing an energy crisis but because our body can't access its stored fuel.
- Sugar cravings are meant to prevent hypoglycemia and motivate us to find easily storable calories.
- Fasting and keto reset your taste buds and rid you from craving sugar.
- Re-conceptualizing hunger in your head can help you not be distraught about it and create new reactive patterns.
- Mindfulness also makes you more aware of your primal urges and conditions you to not eat whatever whenever.

Chapter Seven

Fasting and Freedom

Breaking down food and digesting it requires a lot of energy - Energy, which is the first priority for any organism, and which takes away resources from the brain.

Us humans have managed to develop such large neocortices thanks to eating more nutrient dense foods, such as fatty meat (that ancestral keto diet). Once our body was satisfied, our cognition had the opportunity to flourish and consciousness to reach such high levels.

Also, the anthropologist Dunbar and Aiello have found that there's a significant correlation between relative neocortex size, group size and social grooming in non-human primates[xlviii]. This forced our early ancestors to develop language, which wouldn't have happened, if our brains had stayed small.

We wouldn't have created civilization and started creating art if we had to spend the majority of our time thinking about food. That's why I love the ketogenic diet so much. In combination with intermittent fasting, it removes any feeling of hunger or cravings.

Instead of feeling obligated to eat several meals a day, we should realize that intermittent fasting does us more good than harm and it actually improves the quality of our life.

The Enslaving Effect of Food

During antiquity, the rich folk of Rome and Athens would not eat almost anything during the day and were occupied with other things. At night they would feast like kings and relax. As a child, I remember reading about their grandiose dinner parties from history books. People would have all types of incredible dishes – meat, fish, wild game, fruit, olives, bread, cheese, wine etc. Looking at sculptures and paintings, you can't say that they were fat. Quite the opposite. Most Greeks had a Herculean physique and were not only ripped but also jacked. How did they manage to pull it off? - Intermittent fasting.

Instead of eating during the day, they would feed their slaves instead. Yes, the household servants had constant access to food in the pantry and kitchen. They weren't starving but were being deliberately fed.

Why did the rich feed their slaves? So that they wouldn't get in touch with their primal instincts that gets stimulated by abstinence from food. Their minds remained dull and bodies weary because of being in a constantly fed state. So it happens with caged animals. The lion in a zoo and the lion in the savannah are completely different. One is a sleeping *pussy-cat* – slothful, domesticated, waiting for its next meal. The other one is a *raging beast* – strong, fast, sharp and a king of its realm. Fasting releases adrenaline and increases fat oxidation, that give us more energy and put us into hunting mode. It wakes up the predator within.

How to Break Free

Let's return to the physiology of fasting for a moment.

As you can remember, the 2 governing metabolic states are fed (anabolism) and fasted (catabolism).

<u>Eating stimulates the parasympathetic nervous system, which is the "rest and digest"</u> or "feed and breed" mode. It's meant to make us more calm and relaxed but at the same time slothful.

Ever wonder why you get that post-lunch dip? It's because your body wants to digest food and makes it a priority. The majority of your energy gets allocated to the breakdown and absorption of nutrients. You want to curl up and go to sleep, so that you could store that energy.

On the flip side, **fasting stimulates the sympathetic nervous system – the "fight or flight" response**. The purpose here is to make us more alert by releasing adrenaline and giving us more energy. It's meant to assist us in either catching prey or running away from predators.

Have you ever felt how going hungry sharpens all of your senses? You become more sensitive to the scent and sight of food. Abstinence narrows down your focus and increases your concentration. By default, the reptilian brain makes you search for calories, but if you control the urge with your neocortex, you can direct that heightened attention to anything else.

The catabolic nature of fasting actually stimulates anabolism. Initially it causes damage, which then sets the stage for supercompensation and enhanced cellular growth. It's the same with resistance training – during the workout you're making your muscles weaker which then get stronger during rest.

While fasting, we're causing physiological stress to the body, which conditions our entire organism to handle it better in the future. Without there being a necessity for it, nothing would grow. If we're mostly in a safe environment, we'll soon let our guard down. That's why we should deliberately trigger these responses so that we could maintain our expertise and deadly finesse.

Catabolism stimulates anabolism and *vice versa*. To build new tissue we need to first break the old one down. A shaky foundation won't support any solid structure for long. Hormonal stimulation through intermittent fasting flips the switch in between.

Absence of food and starvation is a signal that makes the body want to maximize food utilization and protein synthesis, making us more efficient with our fuel and causing certain adaptations to occur.

Enter Hormesis

This phenomenon is called *HORMESIS.*

In biology, when you expose an organism to only a very small dose of a lethal or damaging stimuli, such as physical training, cold exposure, heat, sunlight, carb restriction, fermented foods and yes – intermittent fasting, you will get a beneficial response.

The body will always try to maintain a stable core temperature, blood sugar levels and caloric balance. Hormesis disrupts homeostasis - the state of inner equilibrium. Intermittent fasting creates an environment, which requires certain adaptations to take place, so that we could survive. As a result, the organism will then adapt to these new conditions and gets stronger.

But the key notion lies in how much stimulus you're creating. If it's too much for the organism to handle, then it will actually get weaker. What makes a poison deadly is the dosage. That's why after catabolism there needs to be anabolism, and fasting has to be coupled with feasting.

Strategic periods of undereating, followed by overeating will make the body react in a positive way. By adapting to the stress intermittent fasting creates, we will become stronger, healthier and better at burning fat for fuel. It raises the ceiling and power of our homeostasis. Our habitual mode of being will be that much greater.

Seneca, one of the most famous Roman Stoic philosophers, would deliberately practice abstinence from not only food but from all other earthly possessions. He was the richest banker in the city but still would live like a beggar at least one day of the month. For him it was a way of conditioning himself to not be dependent of his abundance and increase his gratitude for what he had. He said: *"Set aside a certain number of days, during which you shall be content with the scantiest and cheapest fare, with coarse and rough dress, saying to yourself the while: "Is this the condition that I feared."*

There's something so admirable about such behavior. It shows that you approach life with open hands and abundance. The scavenger mindset has been completely set aside and there's no scarcity in one's behavior. It also shows bravery and courage of heart. Doing the uncomfortable and getting comfortable in doing so.

Intermittent fasting liberates us. It frees our mind from having to eat so often while at the same time causes a lot of empowering physiological adaptations in the body. The stress response that gets created makes us stronger, better, faster and quicker in our minds. It keeps us alert and on our toes.

In our current environment we don't need extreme survival skills and metabolic efficiencies but they're still invaluable parts of our biology. Ketosis and autophagy don't happen in of themselves but are triggered by the inner conditions of the body. In the presence of elevated insulin and blood glucose levels, fat oxidation and ketone utilization get put to a halt. We don't want to lose touch with our inner beast and primal instinct. We might need it again in the future.

Chapter Takeaway

- Breaking down and digesting food takes up a lot of energy and puts us into the *rest and digest* mode.
- Fasting stimulates the *fight or flight* mode, giving us more energy, increasing our adrenaline and enhancing our focus.

- Hormesis is a biological phenomenon that makes the body adapt to a low-dose harmful stimulus.
- Fasting creates a hormetic response that will increase nutrient partitioning and protein synthesis.

Chapter Eight

The Mitochondria of Your Greatness

It's easy to evaluate one's health and well-being solely on the most evident factors, such as body composition, muscle mass and leanness. However, what's even more important is your functioning on the cellular level. This chapter will talk about how to increase mitochondrial density.

The human body is a bioenergetics machine that needs to be able to produce its own energy. **Mitochondria are the power plants of our cells.** Their primary role is converting calories into energy to produce heat and specifically the molecule *'adenosine triphosphate* (ATP)'. ATP is the currency of our cells used to carry out an array of functions, starting from breathing and ending with sprinting.

Mitochondria are essential parts of cellular metabolism and energy production. They're our inner nuclear power plants that determine how much energy we can produce and at what level we dwell on a daily basis.

***Mitochondrial density* refers to the quality and efficiency of your power plant.** Is the workforce frugal and like a well-oiled machine, or are they lazy, weak and slothful? If the cell's chain of command is led by characters like Homer Simpson, then, rest assured, there's going to be no work done whatsoever and you won't be able to power the entire city of Springfield *i.e.* your body.

Increasing mitochondria involves mitochondrial biogenesis, which creates more nuclear power reactors and is great for spreading the workload. It means that you'll be improving the quality of your reactors, which will translate into more efficient functioning at the expense of lower energy demands. You'll become better and more self-sufficient overall. Running on jet fuel, emanating with fusion power - everything you do will improve.

Given the importance of these small yet powerful cells, it would be natural to want to improve their functioning. The quality of whatever you may be doing will increase because almost everything we do requires some energy to be produced and manufactured.

How to Increase Mitochondrial Density

Increased mitochondrial density is a result of necessity. Simply put, if the body doesn't feel the need to improve the functioning of its nuclear power plant, then it won't do it either. Every function of an organism is there for a reason. So it is with building muscle, intelligence, fat oxidation etc. This means that it occurs in the presence of a stressor that conditions the body to adapt to it by instigating mitochondrial biogenesis.

The necessary component to this is AMPK (*amp-activated protein kinase*), which is an evolutionarily conserved fuel sensor[xlix]. AMPK gets stimulated by situations of cellular energy deprivation, in which the body has to rev up its metabolic processes to keep producing more power. It's a response to an inner crisis, an emergency, that puts the entire organism into higher gear. #CODE_RED

That's quite amazing. In situations of dire need - when there's no readily available fuel source for the body to use - it still finds a way to subsist. Not survival of the strongest but survival of the most self-sufficient and adaptable. However, it's beyond that. We as organic organisms actually thrive in scarcity, as opposed to abundance. Like in the case of mitochondrial biogenesis, we get better and stronger from stressors and thus become antifragile.

Based on that, to increase mitochondrial density, you would have to upregulate the expression of AMPK (for mitochondrial biogenesis) and force your body to improve its functioning *i.e.* become better at bioenergetics (create energy from within).

Ways to Increase Mitochondrial Density

Now to the different strategies to do so. IF and the ketogenic diet are already one of the most potent ways of enhancing mitochondrial density but there are also others that are almost as good. They're going to involve stressors that condition the body as a whole. What ensues are improved fitness, bulletproofed health, enhanced muscles, greater fat burning and cellular efficiency. This is important for you to be able to truly thrive on Keto Fasting. Although you can get a six pack on your stomach, your mitochondria will also get an eight pack, which is a lot cooler.

Strategy #1

Intermittent Fasting

Abstention from food is a stress response that signals the body to maximize nutrient partitioning and speed up protein synthesis. Because of there being no exogenous calories to be found, you'll start producing energy endogenously, meaning from within.

- Fasting increases fat oxidation
- Speeds up the metabolism by 3-14%[l]
- Skyrockets human growth hormone by 1300-2000%[li]!

These 3 are the essential components for mitochondrial enhancement.

As there's no readily available calories to be found from food, the body will release more AMPK and thus has to work harder to maintain energy levels. A state of abstinence forces you to seek a solution to the emergency by shifting into ketosis.

Strategy #2

Nutritional Ketosis

Ketosis increases mitochondrial density because you'll be using fat as your primary fuel source. You'll improve the efficiency of your cellular power plants because of getting fuel directly from your adipose tissue. It's the other side of the coin to fasting and can be accomplished by following a ketogenic diet as well.

Strategy #3

Resistance Training

For your body to induce mitochondrial biogenesis, you have to give it a reason to do so. There needs to be a physiological necessity for becoming a fusion power plant.

Both endurance and strength training increases fatty acid oxidation that instigates an increase in mitochondrial density[lii]. However, there are even other physiological adaptations that occur with lifting weights.

Resistance training is a stimulus for increased protein synthesis and muscle growth. Now why is that good? A part from getting stronger and looking awesome, <u>lean tissue is an amazing predictor of longevity, increased metabolism and bone density.</u>

Having to lift a 400-pound barbell from the floor requires you to contract practically all of the muscle fibers of your body. Your nerve cells and brain neurons will also be firing at the speed of light. During that time, you're producing immense amounts of energy, which needs to be facilitated in some way *i.e.* mitochondrial biogenesis.

During rest, our muscles start to use more fatty acids for fuel. When fat burning increases so does the amount of Uncoupling Protein-3 in our muscles. As little as 15-hours of fasting enhances the gene expression for UP-3 by 5-fold [liii]. In this case we'll be using ketones to feed our lean tissue more effectively.

Strategy #4
High Intensity Interval Training

By the similar token, for your body to adapt, the stimulus has to be great enough. You have to encounter resistance that actually forces you to ramp up its metabolic processes in the first place.

Steady state cardio done over the course of many hours will definitely improve your fat oxidation and thus augment your mitochondria. However, it's not optimal nor the best way to do it.

High intensity interval training (HIIT) is a low volume type of exercise regime that incorporates short bursts of near maximum intensity followed by momentary recovery periods done over the course of just a few minutes. Tabata-like protocols improve both the anaerobic and aerobic fitness at the expense of less time [liv].

Mitochondrial biogenesis will occur already within 24 hours of maximal intensity exercise[lv]. The degree of difficulty is just so intense that HIIT resembles resistance training physiologically with the addition of improved cardiovascular fitness.

You should combine both aerobic exercises as well as resistance training, as it causes significantly greater mitochondrial biogenesis than endurance exercise alone[lvi]. Check out my book Keto Bodybuilding that includes doing resistance training and HIIT on a ketogenic diet.

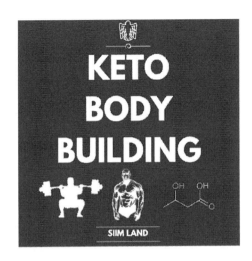

Get it on Amazon.

Strategy #5

Cold Exposure

The key way to prompt AMPK is to make your body enhance its bioenergetic production. So it is with exposure to cold. To maintain homeostasis, a state of inner equilibrium, we'll begin to create our own heat in response to lower temperatures. It increases brown fat[lvii], which speeds up the metabolism and burns energy to produce heat, which doesn't happen with regular white fat[lviii]. Additionally, norepinephrine gets released as well, which is a hormone that boosts your energy, focus, mood and sleep cycles[lix]. It can also trigger neurogenesis, which improves your memory[lx].

One hour of head-out water immersion in water of 14 degrees Celsius increases metabolic rate by 350% [lxi], plasma norepinephrine by 530% and dopamine by 250%.

From the perspective of mitochondrial density, cold exposure puts higher energy demands on the body and increases fat oxidation. But most significantly it teaches the body how to use its own inner furnace to produce heat. It literally makes our mitochondria into power plants of blazing fire.

Strategy #6
Hypoxia

Hypoxia is basically a state of deficient oxygen reaching the tissues. If you're lacking air to breath, then you're having to work extra hard to give the cells of your body enough „prana."

Transient hypoxia stimulates mitochondrial biogenesis in the brain's subcortex [lxii]. *"It can stimulate the expression of PGC-1α and mitochondrial biogenesis in the cardiac myocytes, and this process might provide a potential adaptive mechanism for cardiac myocytes to increase ATP output and minimize hypoxic damage to the heart* [lxiii]*."*

Using training masks for hypoxic training have been found inefficient. For your performance to increase, you would have to train in high altitudes for several weeks at a time [lxiv]. Don't think that looking like Bane will give you superpowers because it won't.

Instead, <u>you can promote mitochondrial density and improve the oxygen flow to your brain by becoming more efficient with your respiratory process.</u> Breathing is the gateway between the conscious and the subconscious mind and can control the autonomic nervous system.

Deep belly breathing stimulates the rest and digest mode, which reduces stress, thus preserving your cells, and reduces the rate of your respiration. Yogis consider breath to be finite, meaning that it's not meant to be wasted, the sooner you'll run out of *prana, you'll* run out of life.

Food for Thought and Mitochondrial Density

The single most effective way of improving the functioning of your cellular power plants is to become a fat burning beast. It upregulates AMPK and turns you into a bioenergetic machine that's capable of always producing its own energy, thus thriving in situations of caloric deprivation.

From the perspective of evolution, adapting to periods of intermittent fasting was one of the driving forces of our cellular biogenesis. Coupled with feasting and eating high fat foods, our neocortex also got bigger at the expense of decreased gut size [lxv].

Fatty acids provide cleaner fuel in the Krebs cycle, as opposed to glucose that by-produces free radicals and advanced glycation end-products, which promote inflammation. Inflammation is the biggest enemy for the mitochondria, every cell within the body, really.

Building mitochondrial density should fundamentally start with nutrition. Food is a source of electrons that influences the body's electromagnetic balance, thus determining bioenergetics.

Eating low-inflammatory ketogenic foods is a sure way of creating a fat-burning engine inside your body. The increased nutrient density will keep you satiated for longer and thus allows you to become more self-sufficient with your own fuel supply, which is key for mitochondrial density.

Maintaining Good Mitochondrial Health

Before you rush out the door to do heavy resistance training, in a fasted state, inside a cyrochamber, while holding your breath, it would be better to first practice *'via negativa.'* It's about deducing the negative, before starting to add in the positive. Losing the activities that are causing mitochondrial degeneration is quintessential, as it doesn't matter how hard you try, if you still have loopholes inside your power plant.

- **Expose yourself to more negative ions.** Negative ions are oxygen atoms with an extra electron and have a wide range of mitochondrial benefits, such as increased sense of well-being, more energy, focus, better respiration and sleep. Naturally, they can be found in environments of sunlight, water and clean air but they can also be generated using ionizing machines.

- **Avoid blue light as much as possible** - it's devastating to mitochondrial health and increases the risk for cancer, neurodegenerative disease, diabetes and obesity. Why? Because it's like glaring directly into the sun – your cells will start burning off their candle from both ends. This is especially important in the evening after sunset. Blue light makes our body think it's still daytime and thus influences specific hormones associated with the circadian rhythms.

- **Adjust to the circadian rhythms.** Day and night cycles trigger specific hormones and physiological process within us. For instance, in the morning we produce more cortisol to wake up. At night time, we increase melotonin, which is the sleep hormone. That's why it's important to avoid blue light after sunset, so that your subconscious mind could rewind and prepare for sleep. More on circadian rhythms and blue light in Chapter Four of Part Two.

- **Drink good water.** The best way would be to get it straight from the source, from a spring with negative ions in it. Tap water is definitely one of the worst options, as fluoride degrades the efficiency of the hypothalamus, which regulates the nervous system, thus influencing cellular functioning as well.

- **Avoid inflammation like wildfire.** Inflammation is correlated with most diseases, as it directly decreases the body's immune system. Don't eat foods high in omega-6 fatty acids, don't use very high temperatures to cook your food, don't eat grain products and processed carbohydrates.

- **Take care of your gut.** On the flip side, a healthy microbiome is the greatest predictor of longevity and health. Eat fibrous leafy green vegetables, use quality fat and protein and add in some fermented foods, such as sauerkraut, pickles, kimchi, kambucha etc. More on having a healthy gut in Chapter One of Part Three.

Chapter Takeaway

- The mitochondria are the power plants of our cells that govern our energy production in everything we do.
- Increasing mitochondrial density involves mitochondrial biogenesis and is facilitated by increased AMPK.
- To increase our mitochondrial density, we can practice many strategies that would make us produce more energy

in situations of cellular energy deprivation. They are intermittent fasting, ketosis, resistance training, HIIT, aerobic cardio, cold exposure and hypoxia, including others.

- To prevent mitochondrial degeneration you would want to expose yourself to negative ions, avoid blue light as much as possible, adjust to the circadian rhythms, drink clean water, reduce inflammation and start taking care of your gut.

Part Two

How to Get It All

This part is structured as follows:

- Chapter One – How to Get into Ketosis
- Chapter Two – How to Know You're in Ketosis
- Chapter Three – How to Choose Your Weapon of Fasting
  - How Long Should You Fast
- Chapter Four – How to Fast and Feast
  - How to Start a Fast
  - How to Break Your Fast
  - How Much Food Should You Eat
  - How to Avoid Refeeding and Overeating
- Chapter Five – How to Fast for an Extended Period of Time
  - How to Fast for 24+ Hours
- Chapter Six – How to Use Exogenous Ketones

Prepare yourself to put all of the knowledge you've learned so far into use. There's just so much value in this information for health, performance and well-being. Let's keep blazing forward with mitochondrial fusion power.

Chapter One

How to Get into Ketosis

To induce ketosis, insulin needs to be suppressed for an extended period of time. As a result, glucagon goes up and starts to empty the liver's glycogen stores.

This is achieved by not eating high glycemic carbohydrates that raise our blood sugar even before we can put them into our mouth. Protein releases insulin as well but to a much lesser degree and does so more steadily. Fat slows down digestion even more. Leafy green vegetables are also safe as the actual amount of sugar in them is small in comparison to their fiber content, which decreases the rate of absorption.

Nutritional ketosis alters our metabolism and makes us use various fuel sources completely differently. Keto adaptation increases the rate at which the body burns saturated fat for fuel and maintains better overall glucose levels.

The macronutrient ratios of the standard ketogenic diet (SKD) are 70-80% fat, 15-25% protein and <5% NET carbs.

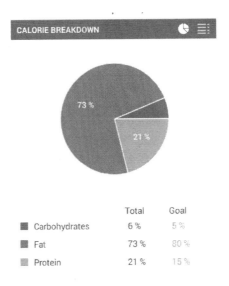

	Total	Goal
■ Carbohydrates	6 %	5 %
■ Fat	73 %	80 %
▦ Protein	21 %	15 %

The List of Foods Eaten on a Ketogenic Diet

Carbohydrates

Total caloric proportion is less than 5%. In total, the carbohydrate intake would be around 30-50 NET grams, fiber not included. The less carbs you eat the faster will ketosis be induced.

Safe sources are fibrous leafy green and cruciferous vegetables, including mushrooms and some nightshade.

Food	Amount	Fat	NET Carbs (g)	Protein (g)
Lettuce, Butterhead	2oz/56 grams	0	0.5	1
Beet Greens	2oz/56 grams	0	0.5	1
Bok Choy	2oz/56 grams	0	0.5	1
Spinach	2oz/56 grams	0	1	1.5
Alfalfa Sprouts	2oz/56 grams	0	1	2
Swiss Chard	2oz/56 grams	0	1	1

Arugula	2oz/56 grams	0	1	1.5
Celery	2oz/56 grams	0	1	0.5
Lettuce	2oz/56 grams	0	1	0.5
Asparagus	2oz/56 grams	0	1	1
Eggplant	2oz/56 grams	0	1	0.5
Mushrooms, White	2oz/56 grams	0	1.5	2
Tomatoes	2oz/56 grams	0	1	0.5

Cauliflower	2oz/56 grams	0	1.5	1
Green Bell Pepper	2oz/56 grams	0	1.5	0.5
Cabbage	2oz/56 grams	0	2	1
Broccoli	2oz/56 grams	0	2	1.5
Green Beans	2oz/56 grams	0	2	1
Brussels Sprouts	2oz/56 grams	0	2.5	1.5
Kale	2oz/56 grams	0	2	2

Food	Amount	Fat (g)	NET Carbs (g)	Protein (g)
Artichoke	2oz/56 grams	0	2.5	2
Kelp	2oz/56 grams	0	3	1
Zucchini	2oz/56 grams	0	2	1

There is also a small variety of fruits and berries you can consume.

Food	Amount	Fat (g)	NET Carbs (g)	Protein (g)
Rhubarb	100 grams	0	2	1
Raspberries	100 grams	0	5	1.5
Blueberries	100 grams	0	10	2

Strawberries	100 grams	0	5	1
Blackberries	100 grams	0	5	1.5

Top 5 recommendations are:

- Spinach
- Kelp
- Broccoli
- Cauliflower
- Cabbage

Protein

Total caloric proportion at about 15-25%. Careful not to consume lean bits without any fat to slow down the absorption, as it might get converted into sugar. The body will always try to find glucose. During the adaptation phase it will happen more easily than later. <u>Pure protein with nothing else will go through gluconeogenesis</u>. Also, egg whites alone will release insulin. Forget about chicken breast and stop separating the yolks. Best stick to the really fatty chunks.

Meat is obviously one of the best sources.

Food	Amount	Fat (g)	NET Carbs (g)	Protein
Pork Chops	100 grams	14	0	24
Chicken Drumstick	1 medium drumstick	8	0	9
Chicken Wing	1 medium drumstick	7	0	8
Bacon	100 grams	42	0	37
Beef, Ground	100 grams	15	0	26
Lamb and Mutton	100 grams	21	0	25
Venison	100 grams	5	0	31

Liver, mammalian, fowl	100 grams	5	4	26
Duck	100 grams	28	0	19
Wild Boar	100 grams	4	0	28

Additionally, fatty fish, such as

Food	Amount	Fat (g)	NET Carbs (g)	Protein
Salmon	100 grams	13	0	20
Sardines	100 grams	13	0	25
Herring	100 grams	9	0	18
Mackerel	100 grams	25	0	19

Anchovies	100 grams	10	0	29
Sprats	100 grams	15	0	20

The best source of protein are probably eggs. They have the entire amino acid profile and are full of omega-3s, DHA, EPA and cholesterol, which is great for the cells and brain. Nutrition of 1 large egg: 5 grams of fat, 1 gram of carbs, 6 grams of protein.

However, some caution needs to be taken. All of those things can't be taken equally. Some pre-packaged products have added sugar in them and under many names (dextrose, glucose, fructose, maltodextrin, xylitol etc.) all of which ought to be avoided for best results.

Top 5 recommendations are:

- Eggs
- Salmon
- Beef
- Pork

- Chicken

Fats

To be honest, there isn't actually a limit to how much fat we should be consuming, unless you're trying to maintain a certain caloric intake. With no carbohydrates in the menu, we need to have another fuel source for the body.

In order to get into ketosis, we need to eat fat and a lot of it. What I'm talking about is adding it on our vegetables, protein, coffee - everywhere.

Food	Amount	Fat (g)	NET Carbs (g)	Protein
Butter	28 grams/1oz	28	0	0
Ghee	28 grams/1oz	28	0	0

Lard	28 grams/1oz	28	0	0
Tallow	28 grams/1oz	28	0	0
Avocado Oil	28 grams/1oz	28	0	0
Cocoa Butter	28 grams/1oz	28	0	0
Coconut Oil	28 grams/1oz	28	0	0
Flaxseed Oil	28 grams/1oz	28	0	0
Macadamia Oil	28 grams/1oz	28	0	0

MCT Oil	28 grams/1oz	28	0	0
Olive Oil	28 grams/1oz	28	0	0
Red Palm Oil	28 grams/1oz	28	0	0
Coconut Cream	28 grams/1oz	10	1	1
Olives	28 grams/1oz	4	0.5	1
Avocados	28 grams/1oz	4	2	1
Coconut Milk	28 grams/1oz	7	1	1

Almond Butter	28 grams/1oz	18	2	7
Brazil Nuts	28 grams/1oz	19	1	4
Heavy Cream, Full Fat	28 grams/1oz	10	1	1
Cheese, Cheddar	28 grams/1oz	9	1	7
Cheese, Blue	28 grams/1oz	8	1	6

All fat isn't good for you. What ought to be avoided are refined vegetable oils and trans fats, such as rapeseed oil, canola oil, margarine etc. They are more inflammatory and actually dangerous for our health. Also, they're biggest reason why saturated fat is considered bad in the first place.

Top 5 recommendations are:

- MCT Oil
- Organic Extra Virgin Coconut Oil
- Extra Virgin Olive Oil
- Premium Avocado Oil
- Grass-Fed Butter

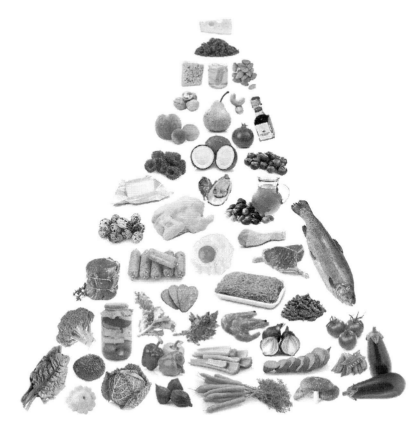

The Real Food Pyramid

Can you already feel yourself better? No more *fat free* yogurts, *zero calorie* sauces, *reduced fat* meats that have lost all of their flavor or other nonsense. It's time to replace turkey bacon with real juicy pork bacon that triggers the *umami* taste of gods.

Chapter Takeaway

- To get into ketosis, you would want to suppress insulin and eat as little carbohydrates as possible. The less carbs – the faster you get into ketosis.
- The macronutrient ratios of SKD are 70-80% fat, 15-20% protein and <5% carbs.
- Eating inflammatory fats is very bad for you and will cause health problems.

Chapter Two

How to Know You're in Ketosis

The process of adaptation takes about 2-3 weeks. At first, you won't be able to experience almost any of the benefits, but will suffer from withdrawal symptoms.

This is called the *"keto flu"* and happens because the body doesn't know how to use fat for fuel. The brain will be screaming for energy and demands glucose. Eating carbs will put a cold halt to inducing ketosis and prevents any metabolic change. You have to persist through it in order to make it.

There's a significant difference between a ketogenic and a low carb diet. One puts you into a state of nutritional ketosis and changes your liver enzymes, whereas the other simply restricts the consumption of carbohydrates while still maintaining a sugar burning metabolism. Staying in this *peripheral zone* won't optimize health nor performance, as you won't be able to get enough energy.

The amount of carbs you can consume while still maintaining ketosis varies between individuals and depends on how insulin sensitive you are.

To get past the initial gauntlet of keto-adaptation you need to have patience and perseverance. The severity of your symptoms depend on how addicted to sugar your body has been before. If you come from the background of the Standard American Diet (SAD, indeed), then it will take you longer than someone who is eating Paleo and already used to less sugar.

During that period, there will be some uncomfortable signs of withdrawal, such as dizziness, fatigue, slight headaches and the feeling of being hit with a club, all of which pass away after a while. If you're lucky, you might not get any of those symptoms and will feel great from the get-go.

This is why the ketogenic diet receives such a bad rep. Because your body is still addicted to sugar, you get tired and lethargic. Your metabolism is geared towards running on glucose and it hasn't been adjusted to burning ketones yet.

To know whether or not you're in ketosis, you can measure your blood ketones using Ketostix. Optimal measurements are between 0,5 and 3,0 mMol-s [lxvi]. The same can be done with a glucometer. If you're fasting blood glucose is under 80 mg/dl and you're not feeling hypoglycemic then you're probably in ketosis. Ketoacidocis occurs over 10 mMol-s, which is quite hard to reach.

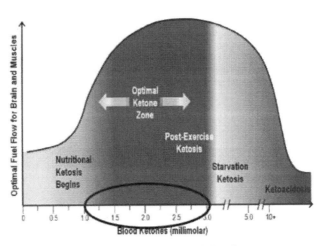

Page 91: The Art and Science of Low Carbohydrate Performance
Jeff S. Volek and Stephen D. Phinney

BLOOD GLUCOSE CHART

Mg/DL	Fasting	After Eating	2-3 hours After Eating
Normal	80-100	170-200	120-140
Impaired Glucose	101-125	190-230	140-160
Diabetic	126+	220-300	200 plus

Additional symptoms during adaptation include:

- **Water weight loss**. Your body will be completely flushed from carbs.

- **Increased thirst**. Because of the same reason. Drink more water than normally.

- *The Keto Breath*. Acetone, the ketone body leaves a metallic taste in your mouth and an acidic or "fruity" smell.

- **Stinky urine**. You're excreting acetone again. Your sweat may also smell.

- **Slight headaches and fatigue**. The brain is in an energy crisis that will be shortly overcome.

- **Lack of appetite**. No hunger because of using fat for fuel.

After adaptation you'll experience:

- No hunger whatsoever.

- Mental clarity.

- High levels of energy at all times.

- Increased endurance.

- Reduced inflammation

- Reduced bloating.

- No sugar cravings.

- Improved sleep.

- Stable blood sugar levels.

- No muscle catabolism.

- Less fatigue during exercise, any other time as well, really.

This is what to expect once you've become fat adapted. You can use Ketostix to measure your progress. But it doesn't necessarily mean you're in ketosis *per se*. Follow your intuition first and foremost.

To be honest, it doesn't matter whether or not you're in ketosis. It's not a magic pill that immediately turns you into a superhuman. Nor is it a badge of honor that you could wear. *"Oh, look at me, I'm precisely in the optimal zone of ketone bodies. Therefore, I'm better than you!"* It doesn't work like that.

Unless you're diabetic or have any other medical condition, you shouldn't worry about getting kicked out of ketosis.

Being fat adapted and burning fat for fuel is a lot more important. This can be achieved by eating low carb as well. However, the initial period of keto adaptation is necessary for these mechanisms to be created in the first place.

For performance benefits, you would want to engrave very deep fat burning pathways and be in ketosis at least for the majority of time. This way you'll be always geared towards being more fuel-efficient and having abundant energy.

We're finished with keto basics. The knowledge you currently possess makes you better off than 90% of the population. Before I hand you the keys to the kingdom, we need to also look into the different ways of doing intermittent fasting.

Chapter Takeaway

- Keto-adaptation can take up to 2-3 weeks.
- During that time, you may experience lethargy, fatigue, brain fog and drowsiness.
- To know whether or not you're in ketosis, you can measure your blood ketones and blood glucose levels.
- The optimal range of blood ketones for nutritional ketosis is 0,5 to 3,0 mMols.

- You have to persist through the adaptation period if you want to reap all of the promised benefits.

Chapter Three

How to Choose Your Weapon of Fasting

If by now you've realized that there are immense benefits to intermittent fasting, you probably want to know when to do it? To be honest, there isn't a definite answer to be given here. Everyone has different lives and time schedules. Actually, it doesn't even matter when, as long as you simply do it in some shape or form. The length of the fast isn't as important either.

Here are a few ways of doing it.

- **24-hour fast.** This is the most basic way. It doesn't even have to mean that you actually go through a day without eating. Simply have dinner in the evening, fast throughout the next day and eat dinner again. This one is also prescribed by the author of *Eat Stop Eat* Brad Pilon. The frequency depends on the person but once or twice a week should be the golden standard. An active person who trains hard should do it less often than a sedentary person. The leaner you are the less you have to fast, but that doesn't mean you can't gain all of the other physiological enhancements from occasional abstinence.

- **16/8 time frame every day.** This is one my favorite strategies, popularized by Martin Berkhan of Leangains. You fast for 16 hours and have a feeding window of 8. Simply skip breakfast and have it during lunch instead. By that time all of the HGH and other hormonal benefits will have reached their peak. It's also the time where our body has managed to digest and remove all of the food and waste from the previous day. In my opinion, we should all be following this. It's an optimal way of eating by consuming food only when it's necessary. We don't even have to be as strict with it. Instead of following 16/8 we can do 14/10, 18/6, 20/4 or whatever fits the situation. The point is to simply reduce the amount of time we spend in a fed state and to be fasting for the majority of the day.

- The Warrior Diet is a fasting protocol created by Ori Hofmekler. The entire concept is based around ancient warrior nations, such as the Spartans and Romans, who would be physically active throughout the day and only eat at night. At daylight they would only get a few bites here and there and would consume a lot of calories in the evening. This diet follows the 20/4 timeframe with one massive meal eaten at dinner.

- **36-hour fasts.** In this case, you abstain from eating anything for 1 entire day + 12 hours. It's not actually that scary as it sounds. You simply have dinner the previous night, don't eat anything in the morning, lunch nor evening, go to bed in a fasted state, wake up the next day, fast a few hours more and start eating again. Going to bed hungry is a scary thing but that's what the majority of the world's population is doing daily. It makes you think more deeply about one's own fortune. If you follow the Fast Formula in Chapter Five you won't even experience any severe hunger.

- **Breakfast and dinner.** As a final resort you can follow the pattern of 50-50, meaning you have breakfast early in the morning, go through the day without eating and have dinner. This way you'll fast for about 8-10 hours and actually do it twice in one 24-hour period. It's not ideal but still better than 6 meals a day. At least you'll be able to not become too dependent of the food and can get the most of the benefits.

There are also approaches like *The 5:2 Diet* and *Alternate Day Fasting*, which include fasting but allow the consumption of about 500 calories on days of abstention. The reason why a limited number of calories are allowed on fast days is to increase compliance. I wouldn't recommend this, because caloric restriction won't allow all of the physiological benefits of fasting to kick in. You want to shock the body and go straight to zero for the greatest effects. Complete abstinence is a much more effective strategy for both your physiology and psychology. Eating something would neglect the entire idea behind fasting, which is to abstain and reset.

Protein Fasting

Another thing to consider is protein fasting. **In a nutshell, you occasionally reduce your daily protein intake dramatically, almost to a zero.** It's a great tool to reduce inflammation, kick-start weight loss and to protect yourself against tumors, cancer and aging.

By doing protein fasting once a week, you're allowing your body to induce *autophagy*. You'll be self-digesting your own tissue. It might seem like you're cannibalizing yourself and starving, but in reality *autophagy* is required to maintain lean body mass and it actually inhibits the breakdown of muscle in adults[lxvii].

It also improves mitochondrial functioning, resulting in better sleep. *Autophagy* is required for healthy brain cell mitochondria[lxviii]. Regular fasting does the trick as well, but regularly limiting your protein intake is another great trick for doing this. If you're not into fasting for over 24 hours as often, then you should still have days of minimal protein intake. This makes your cells find every possible way to recycle proteins endogenously. At the same time, they bind and excrete toxins that are hidden in your cell's cytoplasm[lxix].

How much protein should you eat on these days?

As little as 3 grams of amino acids can inhibit autophagy. MTOR can also be triggered by very little amounts of protein. In total, when you protein fast, your intake should fall between 10-20 grams. Mask it with something to slow down the absorption like fat and fiber and you'll decrease the rate of absorption. Spread your intake throughout the day to not cause a metabolic reaction and you'll be fine for a day.

Being chronically protein deficient is horrible for the brain and body. The trick is to do it intermittently, like with fasting. After skipping protein intake completely (24-hour fast) or reducing your intake close to zero (about 15 grams), you'll supercompensate for that scarcity and increase amino acid utilization.

This makes sense from the perspective of evolution as well, because hunters didn't have slabs of stakes lying around like we see in the supermarket. A woolly mammoth was killed only every once in a while and when that happened it was a feast.

How Long Should I Fast

Fasting is good for you but we should still consider other lifestyle factors. <u>The most important variables are frequency and your current level of leanness</u>. If you decide to fast every day, then you don't need to go any longer than 16 hours. Choosing to do it once or twice a week means you should scale up the intensity and go for the entire 24-hours.

It might seem that the longer the fast – up to 36 hours – the greater the health and disease-prevention benefits. However, that's a double-edged sword. <u>Lean muscle mass is a critical component of longevity, healthy living and being ultimately fit.</u>

The biggest contributing factor to aging is '*sarcopenia*' or muscle loss. Longer fasting doesn't cause almost any muscle catabolism, unlike you might think, but it definitely won't enable you to build or maintain it for long. It will also negatively affect nutrient intake. You won't be able to get in your essential micronutrients – minerals, vitamins and phytochemicals – which may lead to deficiencies.

The leaner and more physically active you are, the less you need to fast.

First of all, there's not much benefit to gain from that frequent abstinence. You'll hit a point of diminishing returns quite quickly after which there are no great advantages.

Secondly, if you want to work-out and keep making progress in your exercise performance, then you simply won't be able to do so as much. Fasting is powerful but good quality nutrition is still the foundation to getting stronger and building healthy muscle.

What I recommend is to have therapeutic water fasts that last for 3-5 days 1-3 times per year, like Dom D'Agostino. You should have a 48 hour fast at least once within 1-3 months and a 24 hour one every 2 weeks.

But it's important to ask yourself: *"why do I want to fast?"* If you're doing it for weight-loss then you should also re-consider your other lifestyle factors, such as diet and training. It's not a quick-fix. *Oh, I'll just eat whatever junk I can find and then fast for a week...* Unless you have over 200 pounds to lose, you don't have to take it to such extremes. Trying to break the 382-day world record doesn't sound like a good idea either.

You can choose your weapon of fasting depending on the situation you're in. If you don't have access to good food or simply feel like skipping a meal, then do the 20 hour fast. At other times you can do less. While travelling it's so easy to do this. You don't want to be consuming all of that processed food sold in airports anyway and IF helps to avoid that effortlessly.

Will It Hurt?

Chances are, if you're used to eating 4-6 meals a day you may find transitioning over to intermittent fasting difficult. Having less frequent meals forces your body to adapt and may take some time until your ketogenic pathways get reinvigorated. You can "ease into it," by starting to eat less often at first and then shortening your feeding window even further. Chapter Four in Part Three gives you a blueprint for the adaptation period in closer detail.

For me, changing my eating schedule happened quickly. First, I started off with the 16/8 approach and pushed my breakfast until 10AM. Dinner was at 6PM and because of that I tended to go to bed hungry. This didn't work for long and I kept pushing my first meal later into the day. It was a lot more sustainable and satisfying, as I got to eat more food and sleep satiated. You have to find out what works for you. It's all one big scientific experimentation, in which the subject of the study is you (n=1).

The best advice I can give you is to simply start. Jump in head first and expect nothing but the best results. You can ease into it and start with skipping breakfast at first, but in my opinion, it's a lot better to simply shock yourself completely. This will wake your metabolism up and tells the liver that it's time to start producing those ketone bodies. That's what I did. I read about IF and after a couple of days started practicing it.

I haven't looked back ever since. The same happened with my first 24- and 48-hour fast. I had always wanted to do it, but had never gotten around to do so. One day I was having dinner and thought to myself: *"what the hell, might as well get it over with."*

The key is to practice IF daily, in some shape or form. Even when you schedule a 24-hour fast but can only make it until the 20-hours, you should still consider it a great success. You don't want your feeding window to oversize the time you spend fasted. 12-12 isn't ideal either. It's better to always be on the negative side of things, if you get my point. This way your body has to always guess whether or not it will get some calories and will have to utilize more fat for fuel.

In the next chapter we're going to look into how we can make fasting super easy and enjoyable.

Chapter Takeaway

- There are many fasting windows you can choose from. It doesn't matter which one you choose as long as you practice IF in some shape or form.

- Protein fasting is a great way to induce autophagy without fasting for several days in a row.
- The leaner and more physically active you are the less you need to fast. Fasting may pose some limitations on your physical performance.
- You should have therapeutic fasts of 3-5 days 1-3 times per year and a 24-hour fast every 2 weeks.

Chapter Four

How to Fast and Feast

Like I said, it doesn't matter what type of intermittent fasting you do as long as you simply do it. To get the most benefit from daily IF, I would recommend you to push your breakfast past noon and spend the majority of the day in an underfed state. Even your first meal should be as low in calories as possible so that your body would remain slightly hungry.

The minimum I would recommend is 14 hours of fasting. 16 is a good point – the perfect balance between autophagy and anabolism - and you don't really have to go any longer than that, if you do it every day. However, occasionally – once or twice a week - going past the 20-hour mark is very empowering for your health.

What I'm going to do now is go through the entire process of a fasting cycle – starting from the last mouthful and ending with how you should break your fast. I'll give you the definite guidelines you should follow and also mistakes you should avoid.

How to Start a Fast

The beginning point of your fast isn't necessarily the last piece of food you put into your mouth at the end of your day. Although you've swallowed it, the nutrients still require some time to be absorbed. It depends on how many calories you've consumed, but usually <u>you only enter a fasted state after about 4-6 hours of not eating</u>. Despite that, for convenience and greater compliance, the best way to quantify the length of your fasts is to begin counting the hours 30 minutes to an hour post-meal.

What you eat lastly has a significant impact on how your fast is going to turn out. Consuming a lot of carbohydrates and raising insulin will leave your blood glucose elevated for a longer period of time, thus slowing down the process by which you enter ketosis. If you eat a low-carb-high-fat meal, then your body will be already slightly *ketotic* as you go to sleep. Then, in the morning, you're more geared towards burning your own fat for fuel.

Sleep Has a Huge Impact

It might seem like this is irrelevant, but I'm going to begin with sleep because it's highly important for maintaining overall health and establishing ketosis.

Sleep is one of the biggest things that gets neglected in our modern wired up lives. It's the time during which our body conducts all of its repair processes. Growth hormone is also released the most during the first few hours of shut-eye at about 11 PM.

Make sure you get about 7-8 hours of sleep a night because anything less will cause too much stress to the body. Sleeping inadequately will lead to insulin resistance, too high blood glucose levels, fatigue, fat accumulation and muscle waste.

The best advice I can give you is to adjust your sleeping schedule to the circadian rhythm. This might not be possible but it's the ideal worth striving towards. The most optimal time to go to bed is at about 10PM. Waking up depends, but cortisol starts raising at about 5-7AM to wake us up naturally.

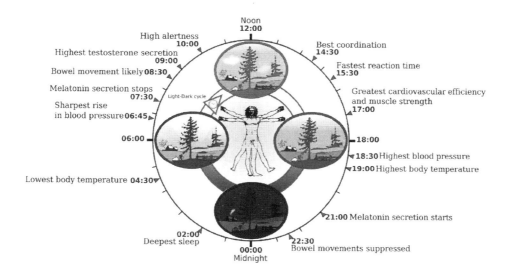

To make sure you get a good night's sleep, you have to block out blue light exposure from your gadgets and technology. It will keep our subconscious mind up and suppresses melatonin, which is the sleep hormone. Start wearing blue light blocking glasses after 8PM and install a software called Flux on your computer.

Unwind your mind and sleep tight. Sleep deprivation will put severe impediments on establishing ketosis and having a good time during fasting.

The Morning of the Fast

After an overnight's fast, your liver glycogen stores will be almost completely emptied. You then rev up ketone production, leading to elevated blood ketone levels.

The most important thing you must do after waking up is to drink some water. Dehydration is another stressor like fasting is and you don't want to overshoot your cortisol right away.

Another thing is electrolyte imbalances. If you don't replenish your sodium during your fast, then you may get headaches, muscle cramps, feel tired and will damage your mitochondria.

What I would recommend you do is add a pinch of either pink Himalayan rock salt or some good quality Celtic sea salt to your cup of aqua. Then mix it all together so that the sodium would dissolve with the water molecules and drink it. This is an amazing way to keep your adrenals in check first thing in the morning. You should add some salt to your water throughout the day, especially if you're doing longer fasts.

Drinking more than adequate amounts of water is very important. Carbs make the body hold onto liquids more easily because of their molecular structure. Once we deprive ourselves from glucose we will flush out a lot of water weight. This is perfectly normal but to prevent any negative consequences of that, we need to increase our hydration.

The recommendation is about 8 cups of water a day but it's not enough on keto. Drink at least 10 cups a day. At the same time, listen to your intuition and also look at the color of your urine. If you're not thirsty, then don't feel obligated to drink more water.

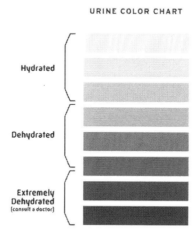

URINE COLOR CHART

What's more, drinking too much water and peeing may make us excrete out our electrolytes more than we consume. That's why you should pay close attention to your urine color and how often you tend to go to the bathroom. If you do it every hour, then dial back on your water intake.

What to Do During Your Fast

You might wonder, what you should do during your fasting window? What you definitely don't want to do is eat food that would put you into a fed state, as this would undermine all of our efforts. Instead, there are several tips and tricks we can use to make our abstinence seem effortless.

Here are the best tips and things to remember that will make fasting incredibly easy.

- **Drink a lot of water.** Most of the time people get hungry not because they need to eat but because they're actually dehydrated. Instead of quitting half-way through, have a glass of water and wait for 15 minutes. Once you've absorbed the *aqua*, the feeling of hunger will go away. Sparkling water is a possibility as the carbonation usually decreases appetite. Also, you don't want an additional stressor on the body and become dehydrated.

- **Non-caloric beverages.** To maintain a fasted state, we need to avoid consuming calories. This doesn't mean that we can't drink some tea or coffee. Don't add any sugar, cream or milk though. Have it black. One thing to remember is to not become dependent of them. Coffee decreases appetite but at the same time dehydrates us. Stick to only a maximum of 2-4 cups a day and resort to it only when hunger kicks in. Don't drink it first thing in the morning either because you want to take advantage of your natural rise of cortisol. Wait a few hours. If you're not hungry then you don't need to cash in on this powerful stimulant. You'll have a back-up card to draw upon once you need it. Green tea gets a green light. Avoid diet-sodas as well despite their non-caloric content. The artificial sweeteners still give rise of insulin, creating a placebo-like fed state. Your body tastes that it has received something sweet but no real nutrients have arrived.

A Quick Side-Note on Coffee

Some people don't preach drinking coffee, especially on a ketogenic diet. The truth is that caffeine releases norepinephrine and can increase blood glucose levels. However, this isn't that big of an issue in healthy people. On the other hand, if you can't seem to get out of bed without having a cup of coffee, then it means that your adrenals are probably burnt out and you should go on a caffeine fast for a few weeks. There's a Bonus Chapter in the end that talks about how to strategically drink coffee without getting addicted or dependent of it.

- **Brush your teeth.** This can help you reduce hunger. There may be some artificial sweeteners in your tooth paste so be wary. You should use it as a last resort or when you don't want to drink coffee. Sugar free chewing gum is fine as well. However, it has some calories in it. Don't eat more than 2-3 pieces. Overall, it refreshes your mouth and makes your breath smell really nice.

- **Apple cider vinegar.** It's mainly used for household and cooking purposes. What you maybe don't know is that it also has powerful health benefits. Lower blood sugar levels, better fat loss and improved symptoms of diabetes. Its biological components are very effective and acidic, that can be good for digestion sometimes. By the same token, it will also destroy bad bacteria in your gut and make you less hungry. You can add it to salads or other food during your feeding window. While fasting, get a glass of warm water and add 1-2 teaspoons of apple cider vinegar. Any more than that may have some unwanted consequences, so don't go overboard. Consume it right away and be done with it. Your body will thank you.

- **Keep your mind busy.** One of the biggest reasons why people eat so often is because they're bored. When I'm fasting I get the majority of my creative endeavors done. While focusing on something else, other than the fact that I'm fasting, then time will pass by without me even noticing that I haven't eaten. If you make a big deal out of it, then you'll inevitably get hungry and groggy. Also, it's a great opportunity to reap the benefits of mental clarity and improved concentration. During those morning hours of fasting my mind is sharper than a knife and can easily cut through any intellectual problem I might come face to face with. Not that I couldn't do it at any other time. It's just that when not having to digest food we can allocate our mental resources to much more important things. Additionally, meditating over it is another great option. Sit down and become mindful of how your body is reacting. It's quite an interesting experience.

- **Move around.** Despite the fact that we're in a fasted state it doesn't mean we should avoid moving our bodies. The initial response might be to preserve energy and stay on the couch. However, doing so would only promote slothfulness and is another way to make a big deal out of fasting. For hunter-gatherers, survival depended on those moments. They wouldn't have got to tell an excuse to their prey that they haven't eaten for a while and would like the animal to voluntarily offer itself to be killed. It doesn't work like that. Instead, they still had to exert themselves during the hunt and had to do so even more than normally. If they would miss an opportunity, then they would have to suffer even longer. Therefore, there was no room for failure. We don't have to go through the same strenuous process. Going for a walk is not just the best way of getting more movement into our day but also gets the mind out of its own rut. Intense training is also an opportunity as the hormonal benefits would be especially evident afterwards. For instance, occasionally I fast for 20 hours, have a hard workout, wait for a few hours and then have my first meal. I'm able to do so because I'm so used to fasting by now and my ketogenic pathways are very deep. What's best is that I don't experience any difference in blood pressure or faintness. That's the way we're supposed to feel even after shortly exercising. It's an incredibly empowering *antifragile* ability.

- **Sleep.** Cortisol is anti-ketogenic and one of the biggest reasons why people aren't able to get into ketosis is their hectic sleep schedule. If you're not sleeping at least 6-8 hours, you may end up with too high blood glucose and cortisol levels. To prevent that, do take the time to have a nice shut-eye. Napping in the afternoon for 30 minutes is also a great way to compensate for lack of sleep and to also make fasting easier. During fasts of 24+ hours, you can also sleep in for longer because it makes the hours pass by faster.

- **Don't make a big deal out of it.** During my first experimental 24 hour fast I realized that the sensation of hunger and weakness is only an illusion. If I thought about the fact that I hadn't been eating for over 20 hours, I immediately began to feel bad. However, by telling myself that it's nothing special everything got better, actually wonderful. It's really an interesting experience. For me, I become more mindful of my blood flow and muscle contraction. During that time one will definitely get more in touch with their body.

- **Write about your experience.** If you're doing fasts that last for longer than a day, then I definitely advise you to document it in some shape or form. It helps you to reflect back on what you may have missed and also takes some pressure off your mind. You can get a notebook or video record yourself.

I've also used some breathing techniques during my fasting, which would reduce hunger and make the entire process more illuminating. Deep nasal breathing into your abdomen stimulates the parasympathetic nervous system and reduces stress. It's a great way to voluntarily control your autonomic nervous system.

Simply inhale deeply, starting from the bottom of your stomach and reaching the top of your lungs. Exhale the same way and do it for a few minutes. This will also massage your intestines and improves digestion.

We should all pay more attention to our breathing, as it's the most direct way our nervous system experiences the world. If we're gasping for air or doing shallow mouth-breathing, then the body will perceive the environment as dangerous, whereas in reality you're safely inside your house. Being mindful of your respiratory process enables you to become aware of what goes on inside you and increases your consciousness.

Additional Therapeutic Measures

While fasting, there are several therapeutic measures that can be taken to enhance the cleansing and detoxification process. Here are a few examples.

- **Anointing, oleation, oil massage**. Massaging the entire body with fragrant medicated oils improves the circulation and detoxification of blood and lymph. It also increases the dumping of waste materials into the gastrointestinal tract for elimination.

- **Castor oil.** An amazing detoxifier because it draws out toxins. Drink one to two tablespoons, flushed down with lemon water, to cleanse the bowels at night before going to sleep, or massage into the abdomen and pelvis to loosen up the bowels. Massaging it into the liver and gall bladder areas will ease purification crises.

- **Clay** is a mineral with a negative ionic charge, which chelates and draws out positively charged acidic toxins. Before you use it soak it in some water for a couple of hours to ionize it properly. If you want to drink it, then mix about a few pinches to a quarter teaspoon of dry powdered clay into a cup of water and let it stand for a while. Clay paste can also be applied to rashes, boils and other skin eruptions to draw out toxins and hasten recovery.

- **Herbal teas.** Different herb teas help the body in cleaning and detoxifying. Since you're already fasting, it's better not to take strongly eliminative or purgative herbs. Use simple and gentle ones, such as lemongrass, chamomile, ginger, dandelion, milk thistle, green and black teas.

- **Enemas and colonics.** Cleansing the colon might seem nasty, but it's an ancient practice and a good idea. On longer fasts, it prevents toxins from old fecal matter from being reabsorbed into the body. Coffee enemas are said to also be very healthy and cleansing. I'm not going to tell you how to do it because it sounds quite bad, but if you're interested, then you should do your own research.

- **Sweating** is another inner body mechanism that excretes toxins. It's our skin's natural response to heat that detoxifies the pours and keeps the blood circulating. We should engage in some sweaty activities on a daily basis, even when we're not fasting. Doing Bikram Yoga and taking a sauna are great ways for conducting these natural purification processes.

Getting used to undereating takes time. Our body adapts to exactly the environment it gets exposed to. Give it frequent eating in conjunction with snacking and you'll be more parasympathetic dominant. Fast and you'll set yourself up for increased resistance to stress and less hunger.

How to Break Your Fast

When you break your fast, the immediate reaction of our urges would be to eat everything in sight. Don't gorge afterwards. If you've mustered enough self-mastery to make it this far, then it shouldn't be a problem to control yourself just a little bit longer. The body needs time to readjust to food and eating a heavy meal right away would put too much stress on the intestines.

Instead, what we need to do is slowly ease into it. **The best way to start off is with a glass of hot lemon water.** The citric acid gets absorbed really quickly and promotes the production of good digestive enzymes in the gut – it gets the juices flowing. This will wake up the intestines and prepares them for the feasting that's to come.

Your first meal should be something small and low-glycemic. This will keep you in a semi-fasted state because of the non-existent rise in blood sugar. Carbohydrate refeeding after fasting causes an abrupt weight gain[lxx]. A spike of insulin will help you shuttle nutrients into your cells but also has some negative side-effects.

No matter what eating window you choose to opt in for, you shouldn't feel the urge to eat any more than 2 meals per day. On a low carb diet, your hunger sensations will be virtually non-existent and you don't need to have breakfast-lunch-dinner with small snacks in between to maintain stable blood sugar levels or keep yourself energized.

After your first fast-breaking meal, you should wait for about 4-6 hours before having your second one. Of course, it all depends yet again on what feeding frame you're following, as you can't eat for an indefinite amount of time on a 20/4 schedule, but try to leave at least leave a few hours in between your courses.

How Much Food Should You Eat?

That would depend yet again on your personal preference. What is your daily caloric allowance? Are you trying to lose weight, build muscle or maintain your current body composition? Whatever the case may be, the general guideline is to eat until satiety.

It also depends on how much intermittent fasting you do and what's your eating window. If your fast lasts for 20 hours, then your first meal should resemble a small mouthful. In the case of 2 meals a day, wherein you abstain from eating for 14-16 hours, you can easily opt in for consuming 50% of your calories with your first meal and 50% in the second. Don't be obsessed by it either – go for 40-60, 30-70, 80-20 – do whatever fits the situation.

What About Insulin?

Does the amount of carbohydrates eaten in a single meal have a significant effect on ketosis? It's true that as little as 5 grams of glucose is enough to cause an insulin response. However, you will almost never eat pure glucose without other macronutrients. The safest of keto carbs, such as green leafy vegetables, already are primarily composed of fiber, which will slow down the digestion process. What's more, fat and protein decrease the rate of absorption even more.

So, if your daily carbohydrate allowance is about 30 grams NET, and you decide to eat them in a single meal, then you don't have a lot to worry about as long as you add a ton of extra fat calories to them.

Carbohydrates are by nature anti-ketogenic, but so is pure protein. Protein by itself, with no other macronutrient, such as egg whites or chicken breast will spike insulin and trigger rapid gluconeogenesis. If you're in a fasted ketotic state and you haven't eaten anything glycemic for a long time, then the body will happily convert any amino acids it can find immediately into glucose. That's why it's not a good idea to eat protein without dripping it into some healthy fats first.

Protein Absorption

It's thought that you can only absorb about 30 grams of protein per meal. In the case of 6 meals a day it might be true but because of the period of underfeeding, our body will be more readily available to use it. What's more is that ketosis reduces muscle catabolism and prevents the loss of lean tissue thanks to the increased utilization of ketones.

Amino acids and some peptides are able to self-regulate their time in the intestines. For example, the digestive hormone CCK can slow down intestinal contractions and speed in response to protein [lxxi]. It gets released in the presence of dietary protein and slows down digestion to absorb all of those nutrients [lxxii].

Our intestines will contract according to the speed at which it can digest food. If they can't handle any more protein, then they won't waste this precious resource away but will store it. After a few moments protein will continue to be absorbed. This happens because the body won't be able to supercompensate without overfeeding itself. It wants to repair the damage and is willing to do whatever it takes to grow.

A single high protein meal can actually be more effective because of that. Intermittent fasting studies show that there is no difference in lean mass gain by consuming 80-100 grams of protein in 4 hours, in comparison to more frequent eating [lxxiii].

Although eating 100 grams of protein in a single meal will elevate insulin, it doesn't mean that you'll get kicked out of ketosis. If you're highly fat-adapted, then the body can actually handle higher amounts of blood glucose without reverting back to a sugar burning engine. You really only need to pay close attention to this during the first weeks of adaptation. After you've established an inner environment that promotes the production and utilization of ketone bodies, your metabolism becomes more resilient towards slight shifts and imbalances in macronutrient ratios.

Your body doesn't have a caloric calculator. It can't go like – *Mr. Anderson...I'm sorry...you've exceeded your daily carb limit and I'm going to have to kick you out of ketosis.* No, this is inconceivable because the state of our physiology and metabolism are in constant flux. We don't burn exactly the same amount of calories every single day and we don't need an exact amount of carbs, protein and fat throughout the year. What's our overall health condition, what are we doing on a daily basis and what are we trying to accomplish are all highly relevant variables that we need to take into account.

Everyone's carb tolerance is different – some highly athletic people can spew out high blood ketones whilst still consuming 100-200 grams of carbs per day, whereas a diabetic will get kicked out of ketosis by even looking at a piece of cake (that placebo insulin is that powerful indeed).

What I've noticed myself is that the longer I've stayed in ketosis, the more carbohydrates my body can handle. This depends on your physical activity levels and degree of insulin sensitivity. If your training consists of very glycolytic exercises – HIIT sprinting, heavy weight lifting – then you can definitely get away with eating about 100 grams of carbs whilst still remaining to be ketotic. Granted, you may get kicked out of ketosis after eating for a few hours but it will probably be re-established by the next morning. You should simply go through a lot of trial and error but always gravitate towards not overdoing it.

Refeeding and Overeating

Why is it that some people gorge themselves after breaking their fast? Are they seriously on the brink of starvation that they can't control themselves? Or are they simply over-eating because they sense food as scarcity and want to eat as much as possible so to not feel empty or dull during their fasting window?

Gorging isn't only a psychological issue but also has physiological reasons that are actually necessary to

overcome. Refeeding syndrome happens mostly when people have been severely malnourished or starved.

To prevent problems in the post-fast refeeding period, you should (1) drink homemade bone broth during extended fasts because of the minerals, salt and electrolytes it provides, (2) take a multivitamin to not get vitamin deficient and (3) do all of your regular activities during fasting, including light exercise (like Yoga and walking) to help maintain your muscle mass and bones. This way you're preventing yourself from creating the purely physical necessity for having to eat obsessively.

Before you eat, take a moment to step back and reflect on the experience. First of all, you realize that fasting isn't a big deal and instead very good for us. Secondly, you should be thankful for having a meal. Most people forget about how fortunate it is to have food around and they become mindless about what they consume.

By doing occasional intermittent fasting every meal becomes more appreciated. Family dinners turn into feasts where eating not only becomes more meaningful but the entire atmosphere improves. Everything, even bland food, becomes tastier as your taste buds have managed to become free from the constantly stimulating effect of refined carbohydrates and sugar.

What's most important, you realize that you don't need to be eating every few hours and can thus accept nothing less than optimal nutrition. Mindless eating in a rush becomes a thing of the past as we teach our body to always have abundant energy readily available.

Chapter Takeaway

- The minimum you would want to fast is 14 hours. Fasting for 16 hours creates a perfect balance between autophagy and anabolism.
- What you eat before beginning your fast has a huge impact on your experience. Having a low-carb meal will make you establish ketosis a lot faster.
- After an overnight's fast you would want to start your morning off with a glass of water with a pinch of sea salt in it. Keep drinking mineralized water throughout the day to prevent de-hydration.

- The key to making fasting enjoyable and effortless is to keep off hunger by keeping your mind busy and strategically drinking non-caloric beverages.
- Break your fast with a warm glass of lemon water to aid the digestion. Your first meal should be small and low glycemic.
- Staying in ketosis for a longer time and being physically more active increases your carb tolerance.
- To not overeat in the post-fasting stage, keep your mineral and sodium intake high by drinking bone broth and taking a multivitamin.

Chapter Five

How to Fast for an Extended Period of Time

Doing IF every day in some shape or form should be the gold standard for everyone to aim for. It doesn't necessarily mean you're going to have to eat only one meal a day if you don't need or want to. Instead, I'm referring to the fact that some people spend their time in a fed state almost 24/7.

If you have your last mouthful of calories of the day at 10PM and have eat again at 7PM, then you've only fasted for virtually 7-9 hours. It doesn't even have to comprise of much food. Even having a dash of milk in your morning coffee will shift your metabolism into a fed state because dairy is highly anabolic and stops all processes of autophagy and the like.

Now, why would you want restrict your eating window in the first place? The reason is that you want to create a buffer zone for your body to do daily maintenance and housekeeping. If you follow the pattern just mentioned, then you'll rarely give your intestines the necessary time to recuperate and rejuvenate their functioning. That's why the minimum you would want to fast every single day is 12-16 hours.

There are many ways you can schedule your fasting and it doesn't matter which option you choose as long as you simply restrict your feeding window. For example, eat only during the hours of 11AM and 7PM. This equates to a perfect daily fast of 16 hours.

Although I love skipping breakfast and don't see any reason for having it almost ever, I also understand that it doesn't work for everyone. Some people really struggle without eating at least something in the morning. There are also cases of serious diabetics who should also consult this with their physician. At the end of the day it doesn't matter which meal you skip – breakfast or dinner – as long as you skip one of them.

Enter Fasting Fury

With that being said, you would also want to occasionally fast for longer than that. This is actually very important for optimal health from a physiological and psychological perspective.

Autophagy is the body's self-digestive mechanism but it's also necessary for the maintenance of lean tissue and brain cells. For basal homeostasis, autophagy is also extremely important for maintaining muscle homeostasis during exercise[lxxiv].

What's more, it's needed for the life-span prolonging effects of caloric restriction.

However, **autophagy can only be triggered after a longer period of abstention.** Although it takes as little as 16 hours of fasting to release this mechanism - after liver glycogen gets depleted - it reaches its peak only after 2 days.

Eating protein will shut down autophagy right away because it stimulates IGF-1 and mTOR, which are highly potent anabolic agents. So you would want to eat nothing at all.

That's why it's essential to sometimes fast for longer than a day. For greater health and a stronger immune system, you should abstain from eating for at least 72 hours 1 to 3 times per year. Doing 24 hour fasts is also a potent refreshment for your organism and can be done more frequently.

How to Fast for 24+ Hours

This chapter will now turn to giving you guidelines on how to first fast for the 24-hour period and then continue doing it for several days. It's thc Fast Formula.

- **The first thing you want to do again is to eat ketogenic before you start fasting**. This will prime your body towards fat burning and makes it easier to adapt to the abstinence of food. As a sugar burner you'll be merely coping with it but on a ketone metabolism you'll be thriving. The faster your glycogen stores get depleted the quicker will autophagy and a deep state of ketosis be induced.

- **Start your day off with by sleeping in for an hour or two.** This will make you already gain a head-start in terms of the time you have to spend fasting.

- **The first thing you should do in the morning is have a cup of salted water**. Add a pinch of sea salt to your glass, stir it so that the sodium crystals would dissolve and drink it. Keep drinking mineralized water throughout the day.

- **Within an hour of waking have your first non-caloric beverage**. You can either make green tea, black tea or any other herbal tea. Sparkling water is also an amazing appetite suppressant. <u>Don't drink coffee yet</u>. You don't want to become dependent of these drinks and use them only when you really feel the need to.

- **Keep yourself busy**. You have to give your mind something else to focus on other than the fact that you're abstaining from food. Take advantage of this heightened focus and mental clarity. What I tend to do is start writing articles, books or make videos on my YouTube channel. You can also read something or simply play games as well – whatever helps you to stay consistent on your fast.

- **Control your environment**. If you see other people around you eating all the time, then your willpower can break and you will give in. Not everyone has the Spartan discipline to look at a piece of cake right in front of their face and not be influenced by it, not even on the cellular level. If you know you have the tendency to give in to temptation, then be strategic about it and take control of your environment in advance. Spend the time alone or with people who aren't eating. Doing it with someone else is also quite supportive and interesting.

- **After 4-6 hours of waking, you can have your first cup of coffee.** Do not add any other substances to it, like sugar, milk or cream – have it black. Don't make it too strong either because you don't want your adrenals to start pumping out too much cortisol. Feel free to skip it all together if you don't have any hunger or desire. Decaffeinated coffee is also great if you're trying to limit your caffeine consumption.

- **Go for a walk.** This very low intensity exercise is great for giving your mind a break but it also increases the utilization of fatty acids. It will actually give you more energy because your body will be converting its own body fat for fuel. Simultaneously, start listening to audiobooks and you'll forget about fasting entirely.

- **Drink apple cider vinegar.** Use it to enhance the cleansing process and push off hunger. It's very good for the intestines and gut digestion. Add 1-2 tablespoons to hot water, squeeze in just a tiny bit of lemon juice and drink it all together. This won't kick you out of a fasted state but you shouldn't do this more than once or twice a day.

- **At dinner drink some bone broth.** If you cook your own broth, then it's a great way to get in some of the essential vitamins and minerals you may become deficient of during extended fasts. The caloric content is so minute that it won't actually kick you out of a fasted state. What's more, the calories come mainly in the form of fat, which has zero effect on insulin and blood glucose levels. If you're fasting for only 24 to 48 hours, then this isn't necessary at all. Chapter Seven in Part Three gives you the recipe for cooking your own homemade bone broth.

- **Use Exogenous Ketones.** Supplemental ketone bodies can promote your ketosis and give you more energy. With that being said, there's a limit to how far you can and should take it. Chapter Six talks about this in closer detail.

- **Consume Branched Chain Amino Acids (BCAAs).** L-Leucine, L-Isoleucine, and L-Valine are grouped together and called BCAAs because of their unique chemical structure. They're essential and have to be derived from diet. In supplemental form they don't have any caloric content but will be metabolized nevertheless. This can help you maintain more muscle mass. Don't exceed one serving per day or consume products with caloric ingredients.

- **Drink herbals teas of decaffeinated coffee.** To suppress hunger in the evening, you can have a cup of chamomile tea, green tea, black tea, jasmine, lemongrass or anything else that doesn't have caloric content. Decaf coffee is perfect as well as long as you don't become too dependent of it. Stick to a maximum of 2-3 cups a day.

How to Use Appetite Suppressants Strategically

What you need to also keep in mind with using appetite suppressants and non-caloric substances is that they will only stray off hunger momentarily.

You're inevitably going to get a slight hunger response in the future. It can happen spontaneously and has nothing to do with how much coffee you consumed beforehand. The difference is that you'll have already cashed in on one of your back-up cards and need to take it to the next level.

Don't cash in on all of your appetite suppressants right away. Instead of drinking coffee, bone broth, having apple cider vinegar and chewing gum all at once, use them one after the other. Start off with the least effective one, such as pure water, then sparkling water, herbal tea and only then have a cup of joe.

You need to ask yourself: Is *the hunger I'm currently experiencing so strong that I have to use one of my tools? Is it worth it?* Because later it may come back biting me in the a#%. Maybe I can ignore it and thus condition myself to have a higher set point of being affected by hunger.

- **Sleep tight.** During your extended fasts, you shouldn't be overly stressed out or too active. Instead, use it as a time to relax and recharge your body. Have a few naps during the day and take it slow. When you go to bed at night you can already count yourself as a victor. The first 24 hours are the most difficult. If you can fall asleep without feeling like your stomach could rip you to shreds, then it's going to be a lot easier from there.

- **Wake up in the morning and repeat.** Follow this cycle for about 3 days. You can definitely push it to a week or even beyond but I do not see any practical reasons nor benefits to it. Unless you have over 200 pounds of extra weight to lose, you don't have to take it that far. Instead, following a well-formulated ketogenic diet and consistently practicing shorter versions of IF will already give you 80% of the results you're after.

If you are aiming for a 24-hour fast, then you don't even have to be fasting exactly 24-hours. Instead, the idea is to eat only once a day and not overdo with your feeding. When you last ate at 7PM the day before, then you can already eat at 6 while still counting it as a 1 day fast. In this case, you would simply break your fast with something easily digestible like hot lemon water or a cup of bone broth and continue on with your regular ketogenic meals.

Doing fasts that last for longer than 24-hours shouldn't be done for the purpose of weight loss but for the medicinal and therapeutic benefits. Of course, you can burn a ton of fat and will induce a severe caloric deficit with it, but you shouldn't think of it as a "get out of jail free card." To actually get the long term changes of a ketogenic diet and habitual intermittent fasting, you would want to focus on building good eating habits that could allow you to sustain optimal health and performance.

However, when you do choose to fast for let's say 3 days, and it's highly advisable you do it 1-3 times a year, you will simply follow the same daily routine. Once you make it to bed at the end of the day you're basically capable of fasting for as long as you'd like to.

After you wake up in the morning, you truly won't feel much different. Over the course of the night, your body will have already depleted its liver glycogen stores and has shifted into mild ketosis. At the 36-hour mark you should start feeling quite good. In fact, if you lay aside the slight feeling of drowsiness, you could say that things are more amazing than ever before.

Most people who I've worked with report having greater mental clarity and heightened focus during extended fasts. Of course, there are still some limitations in terms of performance purely due to the restricted caloric intake, but, when you look at the fact that zero calories are being consumed, then it's quite astonishing how well off your body and mind are during fasting.

My Fasting Story

For instance, at the beginning of this year I took part of a meditation retreat for 4 days. During that time, I fasted and consumed only water, herbal tea and sea salt.

On day 4, I had been fasting almost 100 hours and I felt amazing. Being the biohacker I am, I decided to test my strength at the gym.

It was also the first cold day of the winter with temperatures dropping below minus 15 degrees Celsius and the wind blowing at 20 meters per second. Despite me having not even looked at food for 4 days, my immune system didn't seem to suffer because of it.

At the gym, physical performance did not suffer at all. Of course, there were some limitations on the amount of weight I could lift but, all in all, everything was as good as usually.

When I started squatting, I could still perform at 80% of my maximum, which is quite astonishing, given the circumstances. If I would have wanted to push myself even further, I could have done so easily but I didn't feel the need to do so. What I had already accomplished was more than enough for me.

What Gets at People During Fasting

However, not everyone is going to have a pleasant experience with their fasts. If your metabolism is still quite glucose dependent, then it will nevertheless come across an energy shortage. That crisis can be overcome within 2 days but the difference is definitely there. What's even worse, running on a sugar engine will also induce higher rates of gluconeogenesis and brain fog. To prevent that from happening, you would want to follow a ketogenic diet before you start experimenting with fasts that extend the 24-hour mark. Part Three will teach you exactly how long and when to transition over.

Fasting shouldn't be physically painful. Keep that always in mind. If you get to a point where you literally can't take it any longer and are on the verge of collapse you should end it and have something to eat. It's not meant to be a way to repent our sins or anything the like. Instead, you have to approach it with open hands, accept the limits your body can safely handle currently and then adjust to it accordingly.

The biggest thing that gets at people during fasting is stress and social pressures. High stress environments trigger physiological as well as psychological traumas that create almost unbearable urges to eat. This is the point in which you have to know how well you can handle stressful situations and how much willpower you have. Those who can handle volatility and chaos will have the will to conquer it all, whereas others need to go with the flow.

It also means that you should plan your fasts according to the social milieu you're going to be in. If you know that you're going to go to a big dinner party in a few days, then it wouldn't be the best idea to start fasting now. Likewise, being the only one who abstains from food during the holidays is also a quick route to misery. Eating keto may already cause some people to look strangely at your palate, but to not feel completely alienated, you shouldn't be fasting when everyone else around you is having a good time eating delicious healthy meals.

Some Problems That May Happen Post-Fast

There may be some additional problems you may or may not come across after you break your 24+hour fast.

- **The most immediate issue might be gastrointestinal stress.** Don't rush into it like an animal and take it slow. Readjust to eating one step at a time.
- **Likewise, you may also experience sudden episodes of diarrhea.** Your gut may not be prepared to handle

digesting nutrients right away. It's nothing to worry about but simply something to keep in mind.

- **You may also get fatigued.** Eating can make you feel slothful and tired. This is your body telling you that it's time to wind down and relax because it has already undergone quite a lot of stress during fasting.

- **Getting sick** is the most serious thing that could happen to you. In some cases, your immune system may get suppressed. Not because of fasting itself but because of you being exposed to sickening stimuli in a weakened state, such as the wind, too much cold or other bacteria. Don't go outside with your hair being wet or anything the like.

How Does It Feel Like Going for Several Days Without Eating?

To be honest, there isn't much difference. The deeper you get into ketosis, the less of an effect it will have. Most of the time I feel just the same as I do on a ketogenic menu.

The only thing is that you get more cautious, if that would be the right word to describe it, because of your body wanting to preserve energy. You almost go into a conservation mode in which you're unconsciously trying not to exert yourself. This and having occasional brief hunger that shortly disappears.

The response that gets created is habitual. You have to abstain from eating to a certain extent in some shape or form daily. Every function of an organism is there for a reason. If your muscles don't encounter resistance, then they won't grow. The same thing applies to your ketogenic pathways. What you don't use, you'll lose.

During fasting you feel completely free and liberated from being obliged to eat. After the fasting, you will actually feel more normal than before because your body has undergone thorough housekeeping.

Chapter Takeaway

- To trigger autophagy and seriously rev up its mechanisms, you have to occasionally fast for 24+hours.
- Follow the Fast Formula to make extended fasting effortless.

- Drink bone broth, take exogenous ketones or BCAAs during your fast to promote electrolyte balance, ketone production and the preservation of lean muscle.
- What gets people the most during fasting are social pressures and stressful situations.
- Fasting on a ketogenic diet doesn't feel any different from following the normal keto menu.

Chapter Six

How - Exogenous Ketones

You can also use exogenous ketones during your fast. What are they? Exogenous ketones are nothing else but ketone bodies manufactured into the form of a nutritional supplement, hence the name – originating from an external source.

Most of the products are based on BHB or medium-chain triglycerides (MCTs). The reason for using BHB is that it can be utilized directly by muscle tissue.

When you consume exogenous ketones, you promote the body's production of ketone bodies and provide instant energy that can be put into use faster and more efficiently. Within a few hours, your blood ketone levels will rise and hypothetically you'll be in ketosis, even when you're eating a higher carb diet. This happens because of ingesting pure BHB and MCTs, which to a certain extent circumvents the majority of the beta-oxidation process. Your body doesn't have to be as efficient with ketogenesis or its utilization but will simply get access to a surging source of free fuel.

In a nutshell, exogenous ketones are nutritional supplements that make you more ketotic due to the soaring rise of ketone bodies that the body can readily begin to use as energy. I would imagine them being the ketogenic equivalent of dextrose, which is powdered pure glucose, with the exception that BHB is a much higher quality fuel source that will burn for a lot longer and gives immense energy instantly.

So, you take these exogenous ketones and you'll be in ketosis at a snap? Sounds great and too good to be true. To a degree, this also means that you can remain ketogenic even while consuming a high carb diet. You take the supplement, which raises your blood ketones and decreases blood sugar, while at the same time eating some glucose.

By the same token, it won't put you into ketosis, *per se.* While you're under the influence of the supplement, you'll be in a ketogenic state, which means that the body will be using fat as a viable fuel source. What follows are other adaptive symptoms, like increased energy, suppressed hunger, anti-inflammatory properties, neuroprotection and enhanced mitochondrial density. However, after a while, the effects will begin to diminish and your ketone levels will drop. If you're on a carb based diet, then you won't be in ketosis.

What makes exogenous ketones great is that they enable the body to instantly utilize BHB and fatty acids as fuel. You'll definitely be ketotic, but if you want to get the long term benefits of ketosis then you would still need to follow a well-formulated ketogenic diet.

This manufactured BHB is available in the form of ketone salts and ketone esters. Currently, the supplements that are available for commercial use are all ketone salts, whereas esters are only used in research. Ever since they were introduced in 2014, they've become quite popular. At the moment, there aren't a ton of brands out there. KetoForce, KetoCaNa, Keto OS and Quest's MCT powder are just a few.

My Experience With Exogenous Ketones

Being quite the biohacker and an athlete, I wanted to try out these "miracle supplements" to see how they would affect how I felt and my performance. Therefore, I got access to a sample of Keto OS.

What interests me the most is what's inside the supplement that makes it work.

For Keto OS, the ingredients are:

- Beta-Hydroxybutyrate
- MCT powder
- Natural Flavor (not said what)
- Malic Acid (a natural substance found in fruits and vegetables, produced by the body to convert carbohydrates into energy)
- Ascorbic Acid (Vitamin-C compound)
- Contains milk products and is gluten free.

The macros per 22 g serving are: 110 calories, 7 g fat, 1.4 g sodium, 3 g carbs, of which 2 g sugar (Malic Acid probably) and 1 g protein.

The list of ingredients is quite good and keto-proof, as some poor quality MCT powders (with the exception of Quest) have dextrose in them, which is not ideal.

It's super easy to consume – you simply dissolve it into 15 ounces of water and drink it as a shake. As far as the taste goes, then it's 9.5/10.

This particular sample was Orange Dream and it definitely had a slight citric flavor to it. It's not like a sugary sports drink because of the higher fat content. There's more texture and some nice creaminess to it with a hint of Stevia-like substance. I was very positively pleased.

What I also felt was that it might be actually too sweet and stimulating for my palate. Using the entire packet in only 15 ounces of water would've turned it over the top. Given I've become so sensitive to the taste of sugar due to following a ketogenic diet, I preferred to use half a serving so that I wouldn't explode my taste buds.

What I Experienced

What I anticipated next was how it would affect my energy levels. Before drinking the shake, I had been fasting for about 16 hours and my blood ketones were at 0.9 mmol/L, which is about 80 mg/dl of blood glucose. I was already in decent ketosis where I was usually at.

In the ad, it's said that you'll be in ketosis in less than 59 minutes. So I waited. What I experienced within the first half an hour already was a slight increase of energy. It wasn't much different from having a decent ketogenic meal but the effects were still evident. I wouldn't have been able to run through a wall or anything but I still felt some difference.

After 1.5 hours I checked my ketones again: 1.3 mmol/L, which would've happened by consuming any other keto food as well.

Another thing I wanted to test was my performance. After 3 hours of taking the supplement I started working out. Full body bodyweight resistance training with muscle-ups, weighted chin-ups, handstand push-ups, kettlebell swings and vertical jumps. Up until that point I hadn't still consumed anything else but the shake and was practically in a fasted state. Because of keto-adaptation, I was already used to not being negatively affected by the lack of calories and already do most of my workouts on an empty stomach.

What I'll do give credit for is the feeling of increased mental focus and acuity. My brain had more energy than if I would've purely fasting on water. It masked the perceived feeling of fatigue that may occur sometimes and enabled me to train hard with no regrets. Did I turn into a superhuman and hit personal records left and right? No. I went in, followed my routine and hit the exercises I was supposed to do and progressed in them.

What Exogenous Ketones Would Work Best For

Overall, I was pleasantly pleased with Keto OS. It tastes amazing and definitely delivers you the ketones they promise. The ingredients are fine and you can get some great energy.

Are they a miraculous magical supplement? No, but they're very effective nonetheless. They aren't supposed to be some sort of a superhuman drug either.

When I would compare how I felt on Keto OS with my everyday ketosis then I found no significant difference. If you were to give me a placebo, then I wouldn't tell much difference.

However, there's still an increase in both biomarkers and energy levels. Exogenous ketones will make the 1.0 version of you into 1.1 or 1.2.

Would I be able to get the same results by simply eating keto food or taking MCT oil? Yes, the impact might be small for someone who's already well keto-adapted but it's still there.

Exogenous ketones and Keto OS in particular would work great for people who are not in ketosis and would like to get started. It's also very good for therapeutic use. They increase your ketone levels and may speed up the adaptation process.

However, that would also have to be accompanied by following a ketogenic diet. It would also be useful to use before eating more carbohydrates that would kick you out of ketosis. This will kind of "mask" the carbs beneath the surging rise of BHB.

Exogenous Ketones and the Targeted Ketogenic Diet

Exogenous ketones as a performance enhancing supplement would also work great. Ketones are actually the body's third fuel source – jet fuel – above both carbohydrates and fatty acids.

Now, if you were to combine them with some pre-workout carbs, like in the case of the targeted ketogenic diet, then you would have a much more significant response than if you were to solely follow a high carb diet.

The combination of those 2 would have to resemble *fusion power*, which is generated by the Sun. That's how I feel like when working out on both carbs and ketones.

If you want to read more about the targeted ketogenic diet then get my book Target Keto, in which I tell you exactly what to do and what not to.

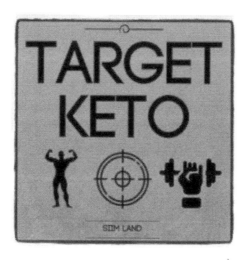

Get Target Keto on Amazon!

Chapter Takeaway

- Exogenous ketones are supplemental ketone bodies that promote your body's ketone production.
- Exogenous ketones give you symptoms of ketosis but it doesn't mean you'll be in ketosis *per se.*
- Using exogenous ketones works best for people wanting to start off with the ketogenic diet.
- Combining pre-workout carbs with exogenous ketone supplements via Target Keto yields a much greater response on performance than following a regular high-carb diet.
- If you're a low carb athlete you definitely have to check out the targeted ketogenic diet and get my book Target Keto.

Part Three

KETO FASTING

This part is structured as follows:

- **Chapter One** – It Starts with the Gut
  - How to Take Care of Your Gut
  - What Changes You Should Make
- **Chapter Two** – Keto Shopping List
  - The Best Food Choices for All Macronutrients
  - Superfoods for Superhumans
- **Chapter Three** – Implementing New Ketogenic Eating Habits
  - Do You Always Have to Be in Ketosis
  - How to Transition Off a Ketogenic Diet
  - The Cyclical Ketogenic Diet
- **Chapter Four** – Adapting to Keto Fasting
  - Phase One: Ditching the Carbs
  - Phase Two: Revving Up the Fasting
  - Phase Three: Going for the Long Haul Fasting
  - Phase Four: Going (Fat-Burning) Beast Mode
- **Chapter Five** – Mistakes to Avoid

Finally, we've arrived at the crux of Keto Fasting. The preceding two parts have laid a solid foundation to this moment. We can now start taking serious action towards becoming the ultimate fat burning beasts.

Chapter One

It Starts with a Healthy Gut

Welcome to Part Three in which I'm going to give you a definite set of guidelines on how to start practicing intermittent fasting on a well-formulated ketogenic diet.

In this chapter, I'm going to outline some of the fundamental changes you should implement to your diet right away and also some habits you should implement. Chapter Four will focus on the adaptation period specifically and its distinct stages.

It Starts with the Gut

Our stomach is the closest point of contact we have with the world and is the most sensitive to external stimulus. What we put into our mouth will travel down our throat into the intestines where it will be used appropriately. If what you swallowed was food, hopefully, your body will release hydrochloric acid (HCA), which begins the digestion process.

Gut integrity and health is associated the most with bodily inflammation levels, which is the greatest predictor of overall health and longevity. Inhabited by millions of bacteria, our microbiome operates like a second brain that is constantly communicating with the rest of the body and sending out signals about what processes to conduct at any given moment.

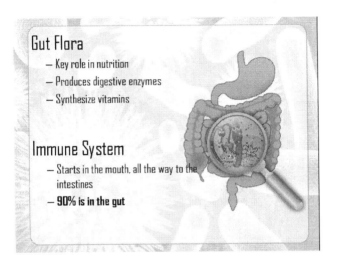

Gut Flora
— Key role in nutrition
— Produces digestive enzymes
— Synthesize vitamins

Immune System
— Starts in the mouth, all the way to the intestines
— **90% is in the gut**

Being inflamed causes joint pain, brain fog and overall slothfulness. 90% of our body's population is non-human and they control our appetite, hormones, metabolism and mood. It's essential to keep our gut clean and happy so that we too could feel great.

The reason why this is so important is that it will determine how well you're going to do on the ketogenic diet. If you neglect your gut, your brain and overall life will suffer.

How to Take Care of Your Gut

Dark leafy greens are excellent sources of fiber, vitamins, enzymes and minerals that feed the good gut microbiome. By adding in excellent sources of fat and protein we're allowing our food to be digested properly and do it with ease without causing inflammation.

On the other hand, if we were to consume refined carbohydrates or whole grains then we will eventually get leaky gut. It's a syndrome in which the phytates and gluten compounds destroy the intestinal walls, allowing the waste to flood our blood stream. As a result, we will suffer all of the diseases we are trying to avoid. Gluten-free might be considered a fad by some, but it's based on real science and solid physiology.

One thing to avoid entirely is the use of antibiotics. If you're taking some, then I advise you to find a better solution because taking these drugs in excessive amounts kill all bacteria, the good and the bad. Also, you will cause gut irritation and excessive stress. Your body will heal itself from almost anything over time. Mostly, our own behavior puts a halt to it. What we can do is just assist the process.

Start eating an anti-inflammatory ketogenic diet. By removing processed food from your menu and eating plenty of healthy vegetables, fat and protein, you're already solving the issue to a great degree.

In addition to that, eating fermented foods is a must. You should eat at least some form of it every day. As weird as it might sound, your plate has to be full of nutrition as well as crawling with bacteria. The best sources are sauerkraut, pickles, kimchi, tempeh, Kombucha, raw milk, raw yogurt and kefir. You can make all of them at home yourself. Commercial products aren't nearly as effective and can have added sugar in them.

Here's How to Make Your Own Sauerkraut:

Ingredients

- o Cabbage
- o An empty jar
- o Salt, pepper, or any other spices you like.

o A food processor.

Preparation

o Use the food processor to shred the cabbage.

o Pack it tightly together with the spices into the jar.

o The released liquid creates its own brining solution.

o Leave the jar open and put a rock or something heavy on top of the cabbage for extra pressure.

o Keep it at room temperature at somewhere with access to air.

o After a few days, the cabbage will have fermented and is ready to be eaten.

What Changes You Should Make

Start taking care of your gut, eat fermented foods and pay more attention to your overall inflammation levels. If you feel worse after eating something, then you probably shouldn't eat it again.

The ketogenic diet works so great because you'll be cleaning your body and resetting it back to its prime-primal functioning. You'll learn more about how you react to different nutrients and how to optimize your intake accordingly. It's not worth it to feel anything less than great.

Here are some additional changes we need to make to start a ketogenic lifestyle.

- **Swap out your pantry.** Get rid of all of your whole grain breads, pastas, cereal, oatmeal, potatoes, fruit, sugar, rice etc. You don't need to have them in your house if you're not going to eat them. At least lose them for the time being. They can only hinder your process. If there are only keto foods around, then you won't even get the thought of wanting to eat carbohydrates. You begin to crave carbs only after you take a bite of them. Pre-empt that in advance like a strategic genius – a recurring mindset to have. If you have family, you should either get them involved or ask them to not tempt you with anti-ketogenic foods.

- **Buy a lot of healthy ketogenic food.** To replace the carbs, go to a supermarket and stack up on some staple nutrients that you'll be consuming from now on. It might seem like keto is overly restrictive but in reality there is quite a lot of variation in the diet. Some of the essential ingredients you should stock up on are.

- o Extra Virgin Olive Oil– Make sure you get it in a dark bottle. You don't want to expose it to sunlight or heat, as it will go rancid and cause oxidative damage. Don't use it to fry at high temperatures either. Use it only as cold dressing.

- o Extra Virgin Coconut Oil – The best fat for cooking is coconut oil because its smoking point is 350°F/175°C. It's also full of medium-chain triglycerides, which are fatty acid chains with medium length bonds and can be quickly converted to energy.

- o Organic Ghee – Ghee is clarified butter that contains naturally *conjugated linoleic acid (*CLA) that reduces cholesterol and inflammation; *butyrate,* which is a short-chain fatty acid that feeds the good gut bacteria; and vitamin A, which is a powerful antioxidant and helps support the immune system. Ghee is pure butterfat that's clarified over an open flame to remove virtually all casein and lactose, resulting in butter with only the best parts of butter.

It's suitable for high heat cooking due to its really high smoking point of 485°F.

o **Frozen vegetables.** To get the most nutrients from your food, you should always try to eat it as fresh as possible. Moments after picking up a vegetable, the micronutrient content begins to diminish. However, refrigerating food will maintain its freshness, as it gets flash-frozen right on the field. Buy a lot of frozen broccoli, cauliflower, kale, Brussels sprouts, green beans, mushrooms, spinach etc.

o **Frozen meat.** The same applies to animal products. You don't want to eat something that has gone rancid or has stayed on the shelf for too long. Exceeding the expiration date won't do you no harm, as the bacteria count will actually increase. However, you should still stock up on some frozen meat. Buy frozen pork chops, chicken thighs, wings, organ meats, fish and beef. If you know a butcher or a farmer, you can also purchase an entire pig or something. Knowing where your food comes from takes full responsibility over your health and nutrition.

- **Stack up on healthy seasoning.**

  o <u>Pink Himalayan Rock Salt</u> – Hydration and electrolyte balance are incredibly important on a ketogenic diet. By ditching carbs, your body will flush out a lot of liquids, which needs to be compensated by drinking more water and increasing your sodium intake. Ordinary table salt is contaminated with unhealthy nitrates. A good quality sea or pink salt also has a higher magnesium content, which is an essential nutrient to have.

  o **Turmeric.** One of the best spices we can use is curcumin or turmeric. It has a lot of medicinal properties, such as anti-inflammatory compounds, increase of antioxidants and brain health. Also, it fights and prevents many diseases, such as Arthritis, Alzheimer's and even cancer. In addition to that, it tastes amazing and can be added to everything. I sprinkle it on all foods and run out quite quickly which is why I also buy it in <u>bulk</u> so that it's cheaper. You can also take a <u>capsule</u>.

- **Ginger.** Continuing on with turmeric's brother. It has almost as much health benefits. In addition to that, it lowers blood sugar levels, fights heart disease, treats chronic indigestion, may reduce menstrual pain for women, lowers cholesterol and heals muscle pain. Once again, bulk or capsule.

- **Cinnamon.** These three create the most important natural spices we should be eating on a daily basis. They're incredibly cheap and easy to come by yet have amazing health as well as performance enhancing benefits. Moreover, they all make food taste amazing. Cinnamon falls into the same category as ginger and turmeric - superfoods, because it truly empowers us. In addition to the same medicinal properties it also increases insulin sensitivity, fights neurodegenerative disease and bacterial infections. What's best, it can be added to not only salty foods but on desserts as well. I even add it to my coffee. The best to use is Ceylon or „true" cinnamon.

- **Calculate your macros.** You don't need to take this to neurotic levels. However, during the initial few weeks of adaptation, you should pay some attention to this. Weigh your food for a few days and follow the ketogenic macronutrient ratios. Counting calories isn't necessary but you should do it as a means of teaching yourself invaluable knowledge about the nutritional qualities of any given food.

- o **Carbs.** The total caloric proportion should be about 5-10% NET, which doesn't include the fiber. This will fall somewhere between 30-50 grams per day. Carb tolerances vary between individuals and you should know where yours lies. The lower your carb intake the faster will ketosis be induced. After the adaptation period you can get away with eating slightly more and don't have to worry about it that much.

- o **Protein.** The ketogenic diet is moderate in protein with 15-25% of total calories. If you're a sedentary person, then your demands will be even less. As a general guideline stick to somewhere between 0.7 to 1.3 grams per pound of lean body mass. If you're a hard-charging athlete, especially a resistance training one, your needs will be higher.

- o **Fat.** The rest of your calories will come from fat, more than 70-80%. Eating more will not hurt your keto-adaptation. However, it's still a source of dense calories. If you're trying to lose weight, then you can't do so by eating at a surplus. You still have to be at a negative energy balance. The reason why keto works so great for this is that the satiety factor will by default make you eat less.

You can also use this free online macro calculator http://keto-calculator.ankerl.com/

Chapter Takeaway

- o Good gut health is the most important thing for health and longevity. Inflammation is the enemy to the mitochondria and brain cells.
- o Eating an anti-inflammatory ketogenic diet and fermented foods is a great way to keep your microbiome happy and well.

- You should stack up on a lot of the ketogenic food staples and seasoning. Buy good quality fat, vegetables and protein.
- Calculate your keto macros and pay closer attention to them during your adaptation period. Afterwards they become less detrimental.

Chapter Two

Keto Shopping List

You're going to have to swap out all of your pantry. Here are the keto-safe groceries for all macronutrients, including their actual caloric content.

Food Source	Calories	Fats (g)	Net Carbs (g)	Protein (g)
Protein				
Bacon, 1 slice (~ 8g), baked	44	3.5	0	2.9
Beef, Sirloin Steak, 1 ounce, broiled	69	4	0	7.7

Beef, Ground, 5% fat, 1 ounce, broiled	44	1.7	0	6.7
Beef, Ground, 15% fat, 1 ounce, broiled	70	4.3	0	7.2
Beef, Ground, 30% fat, 1 ounce, broiled	77	5.1	0	7.1
Beef, Bottom Round, 1 ounce, roasted	56	2.7	0	7.6
Chicken, white meat, 1 ounce	49	1.3	0	8.8
Chicken, dark meat, 1 ounce	58	2.8	0	7.8

Egg, 1 large, 50 g	72	4.8	0.4	6.3
Fish, Raw, Cod, 1 ounce	20	0.1	0	4.3
Fish, Raw, Flounder, 1 ounce	20	0.6	0	3.5
Fish, Raw, Sole, 1 ounce	20	0.6	0	3.5
Fish, Raw, Salmon, 1 ounce	40	1.8	0	5.6
Ham, smoked, 1 ounce	50	2.6	0	6.4
Hot dog, beef, 1 ounce	92	8.5	0.5	3.1
Lamb, ground, 1 ounce, broiled	80	5.6	0	7

Lamb chop, boneless, 1 ounce, broiled	67	3.9	0	7.3
Pork chop, bone-in, 1 ounce, broiled	65	4.1	0	6.7
Pork ribs, ribs, 1 ounce, roasted	102	8.3	0	6.2
Scallops, 1 ounce, steamed	31	0.2	1.5	5.8
Shrimp, 1 ounce, cooked	28	0.1	0	6.8
Tuna, 1 ounce, cooked	52	1.8	0	8.5

Turkey Breast, 1 ounce, roasted	39	0.6	0	8.4
Veal, roasted, 1 ounce	42	1	0	8
Vegetables				
Asparagus, cooked, 1 ounce	6	0.1	0.6	0.7
Avocado, 1 ounce	47	4.4	0.6	0.6
Broccoli, chopped, cooked, 1 ounce	10	0.1	1.1	0.7
Carrots, baby, 1 ounce, raw	10	0	1.5	0.01

Cauliflower, chopped, cooked, 1 ounce	7	0.1	0.5	0.5
Celery, 1 ounce, raw	5	0	0.3	0.7
Cucumber, 1 ounce, raw	4	0	1	0.2
Garlic, 1 clove (3 grams)	4	0	1	0.2
Green beans, cooked, 1 ounce	10	0.1	1.3	0.5
Mushrooms, button, 1 ounce, raw	6	0.2	0.6	0.9
Onion, green, 1 ounce, chopped, raw	9	0	1.3	0.5

Onion, white, 1 ounce, chopped, raw	11	0	2.1	0.3
Bell Pepper, Green, 1 ounce, raw	6	0	0.8	0.2
Pickles, dill, 1 ounce	3	0	0.4	0.2
Romaine lettuce, 1 ounce	5	0.1	0.3	0.4
Butterhead lettuce, 1 ounce	4	0.06	0.3	0.4
Shallots, raw, 1 ounce	20	0	3.9	0.7
Snow peas, 1 ounce, cooked	24	0	2.8	1.5

Spinach, 1 ounce, raw	7	0.1	0.4	0.8
Squash, Acorn, baked, 1 ounce	16	0	2.9	0.3
Squash, Butternut, baked, 1 ounce	11	0	2.1	0.3
Squash, Spaghetti, 1 ounce, cooked	8	0.1	1.4	0.2
Tomato, raw, 1 ounce	5	0	0.8	0.3
Dairy				
Buttermilk, whole, 1 ounce	18	0.9	1.4	0.9

Cheese, Blue, 1 ounce	100	8.2	0.7	6.1
Cheese, Brie, 1 ounce	95	7.9	0.1	5.9
Cheese, Cheddar, 1 ounce	114	9.4	0.4	7.1
Cheese, Colby, 1 ounce	110	9	0.7	6.7
Cheese, Cottage, 2%, 1 ounce	24	0.7	1	3.3
Cheese, Cream, block, 1 ounce	97	9.7	1.1	1.7
Cheese, Feta, 1 ounce	75	6	1.2	4
Cheese, Monterey Jack, 1 ounce	106	8.6	0.2	7

Cheese, Mozzarella, whole milk, 1 oz	85	6.3	0.6	6.3
Cheese, Parmesan, hard, 1 ounce	111	7.3	0.9	10.1
Cheese, Swiss, 1 ounce	108	7.9	1.5	7.6
Cheese, Marscapone, 1 ounce	130	13	1	1
Cream, half-n-half, 1 ounce	39	3.5	1.3	0.9
Cream, heavy, 1 ounce	103	11	0.8	0.6

Cream, Sour, full fat, 1 ounce	55	5.6	0.8	0.6
Milk, whole, 1 ounce	19	1	1.5	1
Milk, 2%, 1 ounce	15	0.6	1.5	1
Milk, skim, 1 ounce	10	0	1.5	1

Nuts and seeds

Almonds, raw, 1 ounce	170	15	3	6
Brazil Nuts, raw, 1 ounce	186	19	1	4
Cashews, raw, 1 ounce	160	13	7	5
Chestnuts, raw, 1 ounce	55	0	13	0

Chia Seeds, raw, 1 ounce	131	10	0	7
Coconut, dried, unsweetened, 1 ounce	65	6	2	1
Flax Seeds, raw, 1 ounce	131	10	0	7
Hazelnuts, raw, 1 ounce	176	17	2	4
Madadamia Nuts, raw, 1 ounce	203	21	2	2
Peanuts, raw, 1 ounce	157	13	3	7
Pecans, raw, 1 ounce	190	20	1	3
Pine Nuts, raw, 1 ounce	189	20	3	4

Pistachios, raw, 1 ounce	158	13	5	6
Pumpkin Seeds, raw, 1 ounce	159	14	1	8
Sesame Seeds, raw, 1 ounce	160	14	4	5
Sunflower Seeds, raw, 1 ounce	150	11	4	3
Walnuts, raw, 1 ounce	185	18	2	4

The Best Food Choices

The foods listed here will be the most nutrient dense sources out there and cover more than one aspect of it. For instance, there has to be more than simply a lot of fat or protein.

Micronutrients and other enzymatic processes have to be also taken into account as the purpose is to get as much benefit with the least of side effects. If the food is packed with vitamins and minerals, then it can be considered optimal.

Variables that are taken into account include nutrient density, appropriate macronutrient ratios, micronutrient content, accessibility, other health benefits and taste.

Protein

On keto, we don't have to stick to lean bits of meat. Actually, we shouldn't either because lean meat by itself will rise our insulin.

By eating only moderate amounts of protein we will maintain ketosis and do not need immense amounts of it. That is actually great. Fatty chunks of meat are the best parts of any animal and hold the most amount of nutrients.

Moreover, we should also incorporate some organ meats at least once a week because they are truly packed with vitamins and minerals.

On a daily basis we can be eating pork chops, bacon, eggs, oily fish, chicken thighs and wings, beef, lamb etc.

However, for most optimal results there are the top 5 sources of protein we would want to focus on.

- Wild-caught oily fish. Salmon, sardines, trout, sprats, anchovies are all great sources of protein but also full of essential fatty acids, such as omega-3s, DHA and EPA. Eating seafood is great for our brain and will allow our cognition to flourish as well.
- Free-range eggs. The same applies to eggs. DHA, EPA are found especially in the yolk. Moreover, that beneficial saturated fat and cholesterol will protect our cell membrane and actually lowers our markers. Probably the number 1 protein source there is because it has the widest amino acid profile covering all of them.
- Grass-fed beef. Meat from animals who have been humanely raised and fed quality food is higher in vitamins and minerals than the industrial counterpart. We do not want to be eating corn-fed cattle as it influences our own biology to a certain degree. You are not what you eat, but what you ate ate.

- **Grass-fed liver.** Organ meats are the most nutritious parts of any animal. All of the vitamins and minerals are found in the liver, bones and kidneys, not the actual tissue.
- **Grass-fed heart.** The same goes to the heart. It's made up of pure protein and rich in essential compounds for optimal nutrient partitioning. We can use different animals, such as beef, chicken, pork or lamb. They actually taste quite amazing once you re-conceptualize it in your head.

Carbohydrates

In order to establish ketosis, we need to restrict our carbohydrate intake significantly. We will not be able to do so by eating starchy tubers, sugar, rice, fruit or pastry.

Despite the fact that we will be eating very low amounts of carbohydrates in the form of calories it does not mean that in the case of food volume. In fact, vegetables make up the majority of our plate visually.

Moreover, for optimal results we want to maximize our fiber intake and nutrient density as well. Wasting our carbohydrate allowance will not be beneficial in the long run. In order to feed our gut microbiome and receive as much micronutrient content as possible, we want to stick to the most optimal sources.

Dark leafy greens have the lowest amount of digestible sugar in comparison to insoluble fiber. They vary in different species and types but are by nature all very similar. Cabbage, cauliflower, broccoli, kale are all different variations of the same phylogeny.

Moreover, celery, cucumber, iceberg lettuce and salad are also simply made up of mostly water and fiber. In order for us to maximize our micronutrient and mineral content, we would want to focus on the top 5.

- o **Sea vegetables.** To overcome the biggest shortcoming of keto, which is thyroid down regulation, we have to eat a lot of seafood. Kelps are rich in iodine and packed with vitamins and minerals. Sea vegetables have high amounts of bioavailable iron and vanadium, the latter of which decreases our body's production of glucose and increases our ability to store starch in the form of glucose.

- **Broccoli.** In addition to its great fiber content, broccoli is probably one of the best foods in the world that fights cancers and tumors. It reduces blood pressure, has anti-aging compounds and improves our immune system. By eating broccoli every single day you are doing your health a huge favor.
- **Spinach.** Yet another anti-inflammatory and cancer fighting vegetable that tastes amazing. It's also rich in potassium which is important for electrolyte balance and overcoming magnesium deficiencies. The antioxidant benefits will also keep our body clean and provide us with more than enough vitamins. In fact, spinach has about 3 times more potassium than bananas, which is considered the go-to fruit for potassium.
- **Kale.** One of the most popular and trendiest vegetables is probably kale. I'm not going to lie to you when I say that it's great but it's not that special in comparison to the other superfoods listed here. Similarly, it fights cancer, inflammation, boosts the immunity and also protects our eyes.

- **Cabbage.** Like any other dark leafy green vegetable, cabbage is as efficient at providing us with the needed vitamins and fiber. It can come in many different variations and colors all of which we should use to maximize our array of nutrients. Bok Choi, Savoy cabbage, red cabbage, chards etc. are all basically the same.

Fats

Last but definitely not least there are the fats which we will be consuming a ton of.

In order to provide our brain the necessary fuel in the absence of carbohydrates, we need to feed the body with a lot of fat that would promote the production of ketones. They are incredibly rich sources of abundant energy and can make every food taste amazing.

It might be difficult to figure out a way to get all of that fat inside our body but by using it to cook our food and spreading it on everything we will be able to get more than enough.

Vegetables are nothing else but a vessel for butter. As they absorb all of that grease we can really create an amazing dish.

The danger with fats is that they tend to oxidize if used improperly. That is why heating some of them is out of the question. To not cause inflammation we need to be very wise with how we use our fats.

Most common sources are lard, butter, coconut oil, olive oil, ghee (clarified butter) etc. But they are also found in olives, avocados, nuts, seeds, cheese, heavy cream careful with the carbohydrate content in them) and of course in meat, fish and eggs. The top 5 are.

> o Grass-Fed Butter. It's the most easily absorbable source of vitamin-A, which is necessary for thyroid and adrenal health. It also contains lauric acid, which treats fundal infections and candida. The antioxidants protect against cell free radical damage and the lecithins are essential for cholesterol metabolism. Moreover, is rich in vitamin D, E, K and has many other benefits. Do not confuse it with its hydrogenated bastard brother margarine, which is actually a vegetable oil and highly inflammatory. Those processed trans-fats are literally lethal, as they cause cellular death. Avoid them like wildfire.

- o Organic Extra Virgin Coconut Oil. One of the healthies sources of fat in the world. It contains fatty acids with powerful medicinal properties and is made up of 90% saturated fat. Because coconut oil contains mostly medium-chain triglycerides, opposed to the long-chain ones, it gets metabolized faster and more efficiently. This provides immediate energy to the brain and circumvents the slow absorption of fat molecules.

- o MCT Oil. The liquidized form of coconut oil. If you want to speed up your keto adaptation, then using MCTs is a must. Being one of the most powerful sources of calories imaginable, it basically operates like liquid glucose. It gets absorbed and converted into energy extremely fast. In fact, it might happen too quickly as too much of it can cause diarrhea.

- o Extra Virgin Olive Oil **and olives.** A staple of the Mediterranean diet, they have anti-inflammatory substances and protect the heart against cardiovascular disease. Beware not to heat it, as the fatty acids in olive oil can oxidize and cause cellular damage if consumed. It's best we use it as cold dressing instead.

- ○ **Avocados.** Loaded with heart-healthy monounsaturated fatty acids they also contain more potassium than bananas. Eating avocados lowers cholesterol, triglyceride levels and protects against cancer. It can also help you absorb nutrients from other plant foods. The saying: *an apple a day keeps the doctor away* should be replaced with *an avocado a day.*

These are the top 5 sources of every macronutrient we should be eating for the majority of our time. The purpose is to maximize micronutrient content, beneficial effects and nutrient partitioning from our food. This is a list of true superfoods that empower us and enable us to reach optimal health, improve our performance and longevity.

Superfoods for Superhumans

On the other hand, there are also some additional "superfoods" we can consume. They are slightly less conventional and harder to find. Nevertheless, they are incredibly empowering and take it to the next level. Occasionally using them will yield great results.

First off, it's important to understand what we mean by "superfoods." Broccoli and turmeric fight cancer and reduce inflammation, eggs and salmon have omega-3s and DHA and can be considered as such. Because of the benefits we get from them, they are already a part of the list. However, they lack that one last push that would twist the entire thing over the top.

A superfood for a superhuman would have to be something that transcends their health and performance past our normal capacities and reach levels of post-optimal wellbeing.

Here's a list of some TRUE superfoods.

- **Blueberries.** Why? They're full of phytonutrients, that neutralize free radicals. The high antioxidant content also protects against cancer and reduces the effects of Alzheimer's and Parkinson's disease. They're brain food that improves cognitive functioning and memory. At the same time, it reduces the risk of heart disease and muscle damage from exercise.

- **Cacao.** Not hot chocolate, but raw cacao nibs. They can improve your memory, reduce heart disease, increase fat oxidation, boost immunity and grant a lot of energy. The Incas considered it the drink of the gods. Raw cacao contains 20 times more antioxidants than blueberries and 119 times more than bananas – there's your micronutrient bomb. Processed chocolate is made with roasted cocoa, milk, sugar and trans fats that block the absorption of antioxidants. Organic more than 80% dark chocolate can have the same benefits as raw cacao.

- Chia seeds. A very popular superfood because of its nutrient density and easy digestion. Aztec warriors ate chia seeds before battle for high energy and endurance. A spoonful was said to sustain them for 24 hours. In the Mayan language, "Chia" means "strength." These seeds are rich in fiber, omega-3s, protein, vitamins and minerals, such as copper, zinc and potassium. They will boost our metabolism, protect against heart disease, build muscle and increase fat burning. To get the most nutrition, you have to soak them in water for a few hours before consumption.

- **Algae.** It's a complex superfood that can be found in green, blue-green or brown seaweed. The health benefits are quite amazing: stronger immune system, increased white blood cell count and better gut flora. Blue-green algae like Chlorella or Spirulina is a source of vitamin B12 and 22 other amino acids. Brown algae contains *Fuxoaxanthin* that promotes fat burning.

- Bee pollen. Made by honeybees, it is one of the most nourishing foods Mother Nature can provide us with, as it contains almost all of the essential nutrients needed by humans. It's rich in amino acids, vitamins, including B-complex, and folic acid. Bee pollen is richer in protein than any animal source and half of it is directly used by the body. One teaspoon consists of over 2,5 billion (that's 9 zero digits – 2 500 000 000) flower pollen grains. Talk about micronutrient density. The benefits include: enhanced energy, smoother skin, high amounts of antioxidants, allergy reduction, improved digestion, stronger immune and cardiovascular system.

Chapter Takeaway

- Micronutrient content is a lot more important for health and performance than macros.
- You should eat mostly the top 5 foods for each macronutrient group.
- Occasionally eat some superfoods for superhuman vitality. They're worth it.

Chapter Three

New Ketogenic Eating Habits

A sustainable shift towards keto fasting needs to also be accompanied by changing some of your eating habits. The purpose isn't to restrict yourself from doing certain things but to create new patterns of behavior that would improve your relationship with food for the better and turn yourself into the YOU+ version of yourself.

What's the secret to sticking to healthy habits as a long term thing? It's not about pushing through with sheer willpower, although you need some discipline initially. Instead, you simply have to create yourself a certain set of rules that you will begin to follow from now on. Come hell or high water...

The first rules you should make immediately are:

- No more eating 3-5 times per day
- No more snacking on the run
- No more eating in bed
- No more turning a blind eye to unscheduled cheats
- No more binging or emotional eating

- Always savor your first bite after a fast
- Don't eat until you've completely prepared your dish

Your own individual preferences may require a different set of rules and these are only a few examples. At the same time, don't get too attached to your rules either because that marks the point of you being controlled by them not the other way around. You want to maintain this elusive balance between being disciplined and spontaneous. However, if you want to truly reap all of the promised benefits of keto then you must stay consistent and focused on the path.

Realize this: your habits and taste preferences have nothing to do with who you truly are. They are simply habitual patterns of thinking and behaving that stem from your past condition and history. If you were to grow up in a different environment and get exposed to other stimuli you would value other things.

Why do you think some people report getting incredible enjoyment out of natural whole foods, such as raw cabbage, whereas others need to add a ton of salt and sugar to their dish in order to get any sensation from it?

Human beings adapt to ketosis, hormesis and fasting but we also get used to the stimuli we get exposed to the most. It's homeostasis in work again. Whatever seems appealing to you is purely subjective and isn't necessarily beneficial. In this case, it can be adjusted and changed for the better. You'll be happier and more efficient of a human being if you do this.

The Key to Habit Change

Breaking bad habits is difficult at first because we are stuck inside them. <u>What you need to do is replace one habit with another.</u> Replace the habit of always having dessert after dinner with the habit of drinking herbal tea. It's a skill that allows you to constantly break up patterns that don't serve you and adjust your behavior in a way that contributes to your greater cause. Eventually, you'll be liberated from them completely and can thus truly live a fulfilling life the way you like it.

Do You Always Have to Be in Ketosis?

We're living in an anti-ketogenic world. Massive amounts of carbohydrates and trans fats are surrounding us everywhere – they're in our grocery stores, coffee shops, office space, pantries and kitchen cupboards. The Western cuisine is built up on a SAD template that promotes inflammation, lethargy and poor health.

Nevertheless, we as people are living members of that culture and not all carbs are inherently damaging or bad. Low carb fanatics are making the same mistake as the *carboholics* did in the past by blaming it all on one single macronutrient.

In reality, the reason for the poor health condition of so many people isn't this thing or the other. It's the culmination and combination of several factors that create a hectic environment in our inner biology. On top of that, our outer world is also unforgiving and as a result our biology will suffer.

Although ketosis alleviates and cures a lot of the symptoms and diseases people are struggling with, it's not a miracle drug nor the end-all-be-all. <u>The fact of the matter is that you don't have to nor should be in ketosis 24/7 for the remainder of your life.</u>

Getting into ketosis the first time may take a week or two, depending on your degree of carbohydrate tolerance. It's true that the longer you stay in it, the better you'll start to feel. Your mental acuity and energy levels will be on point for the majority of the time. What's more, after proper fat adaptation, your physical performance will also get enhanced.

Nevertheless, you may come across various situations wherein you don't have the means or desire to follow a ketogenic diet. Maybe you choose to become a professional athlete who's in need of more glycogen, maybe it's the holidays and you want to eat some cake, maybe you're in a meditation retreat where people eat vegan – whatever it might be.

Getting off keto isn't detrimental nor difficult. <u>Intermittent fasting is, in my opinion, a much more important strategy for health.</u> Also, you can actually stay in ketosis to a certain degree as long as you practice IF. You won't lose your fat burning pathways anyway, as long as you won't start eating copious amounts of simple sugars and refined carbs SAD style.

How to Transition Off a Ketogenic Diet

The only problem with getting off keto is that you may experience an abrupt weight gain. After you go low carb, your body will get flushed from glucose and begins to hold onto less water. As a result, you will seemingly lose a few pounds almost at an instant. However, this isn't actual fat loss but simply liquid retention.

Once you start eating carbs again, your muscles will re-absorb those carbohydrate molecules and your body will become more "fuller." It has nothing to do with ketosis – it's just the natural tendency of our body to react to certain nutrients. For instance, eating a lot of sodium will also make you retain more water. When on keto this is less so because you hold less glycogen to begin with, so it's all depends on many variables.

To prevent yourself from gaining a lot of weight after getting off a keto diet, you would want to ease out of it slowly. Rather than starting to binge on starchy tubers, pasta and bread, you would want to re-introduce larger quantities of carbs over time.

Getting Off Keto

- **During the first week off from keto, you would want to eat around 100 grams of carbs mainly from fibrous tubers and vegetables,** such as carrots, beetroot and berries. Do keep eating the low carb cruciferous veggies because their micronutrient properties and anticancerous compounds are quite amazing. Just don't eat a lot of starch yet.

- **The second week can be more liberal in terms of what you eat.** Start adding a potato or a cup of rice to your dinner on days you're most physically active. Don't overdo it either if you want to maintain at least semi-ketosis for at least some parts of the day. In total, your daily carb intake would fall somewhere between 100 and 200 grams.

- **Third week in, eat moderate carb.** In this stage you can eat starchy tubers, fruit and grains as long as you keep yourself physically active in some degree. I wouldn't recommend anyone but professional athletes to eat a high carb diet because of blood sugar reasons. Despite you being off keto, the key to greater health is still controlling insulin. How many carbs you can get away with depends on your level of leanness, insulin sensitivity, how much you train and how much muscle mass you have. Generally, 200 to 300 grams per day should be the upper limit if you want to be in mild-ketosis while fasting in the morning.

- **Keep practicing IF daily**. The beauty of intermittent fasting is that it works with every diet and it doesn't require you to be manically obsessed by what you eat. Although it works best and is the healthiest on a keto, you can and should practice it in some shape or form almost every day. Don't revert back to eating 3-5 small meals a day.

- **Eat carbs strategically.** By the same token, you don't want to be eating carbohydrates randomly. Your first meal of the day with which you break your fast should still be low glycemic and ketogenic. This will sustain a fasted state and keeps your fat burning pathways engrained within you at least to a certain degree. The best time to eat carbs is post-workout when your muscle glycogen stores are already empty and ready to absorb some fuel.

Herein we can turn to the cyclical ketogenic diet (CKD). This works great for people who want to stay on keto but also would like to have carb cheat days every now and then.

Enter The Cyclical Ketogenic Diet

In a nutshell – you eat keto for a given period and then have massive refeeds with a lot of carbohydrates.

The CKD can be structured anyway you like. You can either have refeeds for one day of the week or once a month. Maybe you only choose to have carbs only a handful times of the year – again, whatever suits the situation. By incorporating IF and keto, you can be very flexible with your eating and don't have to worry about suffering almost any negative consequences of indulgence.

The common CKD involves 1-2 days of refeeding after exhaustive exercise. On the first day you eat only high glycemic carbohydrates and on the second you eat low glycemic ones. This overcomes the limiting time-factor of glycogen re-synthesis.

However, in my own experience, I don't see any significant benefit to this. If you're a natural athlete, then you don't need to lengthen your refeed to any more than one day - one massive meal, really. This will benefit your health and keto adaptation that much more.

You eat ketogenic throughout the week and then, on one afternoon in the weekend, you begin to feast on some carbohydrates until bedtime. It's more sustainable this way and, unless you have a competitive reason or an upcoming athletic event, you don't need to carb load for several days. I call it the Keto Cycle.

Here's How to Do the Keto Cycle

- First, get fully keto-adapted. Eat low carb for about 2-3 weeks before trying anything.

- Then, schedule a re-feed day on one of your harder training sessions.

- While in a fasted state, have a workout in the afternoon that focuses on higher reps. This will deplete your glycogen stores and primes your muscles to be hungrier for carbs.

- Throw in some HIIT as well, if you want to increase the effects of supercompensation. This is the time to go all out, as you'll be refeeding later.

- After your workout, at about 4-5 PM, break your fast with something high glycemic that spikes your insulin. The best foods for this are white rice, white potatoes, whey protein shakes with dextrose, extra ripe bananas with dark spots on them or honey.

- Let your insulin rise and spend the rest of the night refeeding on massive quantities of carbohydrates. Eat moderate protein, this time only the lean bits, such as whitefish, cottage cheese and chicken breast. Avoid too much fats (eat about 30 grams), because it can be stored directly as fat with elevated levels of insulin.

There's a lot more that goes into this and a lot could go wrong. If you're interested in how to do the cyclical ketogenic diet in closer detail, then you should definitely get my book called Keto Cycle. It teaches you how to get your cake and eat it too.

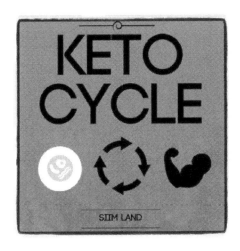

Get it on Amazon!

Chapter Takeaway

- The key to sticking to good habits is creating a set of rules for you to follow.
- Your habits and taste preferences are not who you truly are but merely the conditioning you've received from your environment. They can be changed for the better.
- Break bad habits by replacing them with a good one.
- To not experience an abrupt weight gain while getting off a ketogenic diet, you would want to slowly ease out of it by bringing carbs back in gradually.
- The cyclical ketogenic diet involves eating keto for a certain period and then re-feeding on massive amounts of carbs. This works great for body composition athletes.
- If you want to learn all the nitty-gritty of CKD, you should definitely get my book Keto Cycle.

Chapter Four

Adapting to Keto Fasting

So far, I've bestowed you with a ton of invaluable knowledge about the ketogenic diet and intermittent fasting. The combination of these two strategies is truly remarkable and powerful because you'll turn your body into a self-sufficient powerhouse with abundant vitality and energy.

Although I've already given you so much information that it would be easy to start following your own nutritional plan, I'm now going to give you an exact blueprint for the adaptation period.

Keep in mind that nutrition is highly individualized and context dependent and this is just a general attempt to give you a one-size-fits-all solution. I cannot possibly know your medical history, body composition or goals.

If, however, you feel like you do need some additional assistance in coming up with a diet plan, then feel free to contact me via e-mail at siimlandd@gmail.com for some personal coaching.

Phase One

Ditching the Carbs

The first step towards becoming a fat burning machine is to go on a low carb diet.

Although the quickest and easiest way to get into ketosis is to fast for 3-5 days, I wouldn't recommend you doing it in the beginning.

If you're used to eating, let's say 30-50% of your calories from carbohydrates, which amounts to roughly 150-250 grams for an average weighing adult, then your body won't handle fasting very well. Don't get me wrong, you would get into deep ketosis and would feel quite good but you would still initially suffer higher rates of gluconeogenesis.

Before you start experimenting with extended fasts, you would want to be already quite good at burning your own body fat for fuel. This can be accomplished by following a well-formulated ketogenic diet for at least 2 weeks.

However, it doesn't mean that you can't be practicing IF. Instead, you would still stick to the daily restricted feeding window and abstain from food outside of it.

The perfect balance for this is the 16-8 frame, in which you eat only 2 meals a day – lunch and dinner/ breakfast and an afternoon meal/ dinner and brunch. You don't have to be neurotic about it but simply try to spend the majority of your waking hours in a fasted state.

The foods eaten would follow the standard ketogenic diet macronutrient ratios: 70-80% fat, 15-20% protein and <5% carbohydrates (30-50 grams NET).

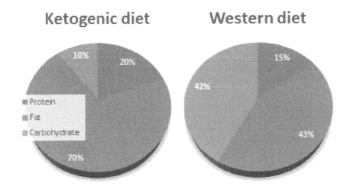

Whenever you break your fast, start off with a small low glycemic dish that doesn't have a lot of caloric content. My go-to "breakfast" at that time was 3-4 eggs, 1 cup of spinach, 2

tbsp of butter and 1-2 Brazil nuts. This amounted in total under 500 calories and kept me satiated until the evening. The recipe is in Chapter Six.

Phase Two
Revving Up the Fasting

After about 1,5 to 2 weeks, you'll be already quite ketotic. As long as you stay under your daily carb allowance, you will have probably depleted your glycogen stores completely. In reaction, your blood stream will have elevated ketone levels. However, it doesn't mean you're utilizing them successfully.

Having high blood ketones doesn't necessarily mean that you're in ketosis. This needs to be accompanied by a decreased level of blood glucose as well.

One of the surest ways of lowering blood sugar is through fasting. Eating low carb does so as well, but some people may struggle because of pre-diabetes or excessive cortisol floating about.

You would want to incorporate longer fasts for medicinal and therapeutic benefits anyway, so this is the perfect time for you to have your first 24-hour fast. Follow the guidelines given in Chapter Five of Part Two and you'll be striving.

How often should you have a one day fast?

That would depend on several variables, but no more than once or twice a week. The minimum should also be once or twice a month.

You can also increase your fasting window and eat on a 20/4 schedule. This works perfectly fine and is great for rapid weight loss. If you're aiming for caloric maintenance, then it's also a very comfortable way of eating.

Phase Three
Going for the Long Haul

Now, after you've had at least two to three 24-hour fasts and have been eating keto for more than a month, you can begin experimenting with exceeding the one day mark.

Before you start off with crazy 5 day fasts during which you exercise and not sleep much, you would want to try out fasting for 40-48 hours. Going to bed without having eaten anything and then waking up to continue your abstinence is a physiological stressor to which your body can easily adapt. However, it will also be a psychological shock to your mind and you may not have the willpower to follow through.

Instead of making it a grind, you can simply fast for as long as you feel comfortable with. It doesn't have to be a struggle and it mustn't be painful. If you've followed the previous stages then it shouldn't be difficult to go without eating for 48 hours. Know your limits but, nevertheless, always try to exceed them.

To be honest, after you complete your first 2 day fast you're all set for fasting as long as you'd like to. Of course, there are limits to how far you should take it but getting past the first 24-hours is the only real difficult part. Once you cross that milestone, you'll decrease gluconeogenesis thanks to the surge in growth hormone and soaring amounts of ketone bodies.

It's also counterproductive to stop fasting at that point. You've made it past the most difficult point and are only starting to reap the greatest benefits. Why not go any further when you've already made it this far?

The way you feel between day 3 and day 6 isn't that different. It's all accompanied by stable blood sugar and energy so there isn't many significant changes you can recognize within your body.

However, you may experience some slight discomforts and signs of fatigue. This is a sign that you should increase your sodium intake. <u>Lethargy, muscle cramps and hypoglycemia have mostly to do with an electrolyte imbalance not starvation</u>. It may also mean that you should lay down for a moment and take it slow.

If these signs subsist for more than an hour, you should definitely stop fasting and rest. Keep experimenting with 2-3 of these 48 hour fasts before you move on.

Phase Four
Going (Fat Burning) Beast Mode

Doing intermittent fasting on a ketogenic diet puts your body in a prime-primal physiological state in which you have access to abundant energy endogenously. This was the mechanism that allowed out species to thrive at times of scarcity in the past, and in the present helps us to expand on our human potential.

If you're capable of going through an entire day without eating nor feeling hunger pains, then you can also fast for several days with ease. This marks the point, in which you can fast for 3+ days while maintaining your sanity and productivity. Usually, it takes about a few months before you can truly tap into your fat burning beast.

None of us can really comprehend how far we can take our bodies. We're actually a lot stronger, resilient, smarter and faster than we think. Practicing IF and keto helps me to remember that deep inside me there's my primal aspect that's simply lying there dormant – waiting to be awakened. Whenever that happens, let's say after having fasted for many days and then hitting the gym to hit near personal records, I feel truly empowered and unstoppable.

With Great Power Comes Great Responsibility

Although you now have the potential to not eat for a week and not give a damn, you also need to ask yourself this: *"Why am I doing this? Do I need to be fasting for so long so often? Would my life be better if I ate just one meal a day or will I get 80% of the results I'm after by having just two?"* These questions help you understand your reasons and assist you in determining how frequently you should fast.

Because IF is just so comfortable and enjoyable, it's easy to start over-doing it. If you've reached your goal weight, then you don't have to be nearly as strict with this. I have to keep re-iterating myself for many times but it doesn't matter how long you fast, as long as you simply do it in some shape or form.

If you begin to show signs of too much fasting, such as muscle loss, exhaustion, overeating, cramps, mood swings and shivering, then you should dial down for a little bit and eat slightly more for a few days. You want to do this as a long term thing and not burn yourself out completely.

Chapter Takeaway

- To make your adaptation period as enjoyable as possible, start off with eating a ketogenic diet and doing 16/8 hour fasting daily.
- After about 2 weeks, start incorporating 24-hour fasts once a week and move on from there.
- If you've been eating keto for about a month and have had a few 24-hour fasts, schedule your first 2 day fast.

- Have a 48 hour fast once within 2-3 months.

- You should go for 3+ day fasts only after having had two 48 fasts.

- Fast for 3-5 days 2-3 times a year.

Chapter Five

Mistakes to Avoid

Going through the adaptation period is difficult but highly rewarding afterwards. Having done it quite a few times myself I can tell that it gets easier the more you do it. The more your body knows how to use fat for fuel the less side effects you'll have. My own experiments with ketosis have taught me a lot about nutrition and how to become more efficient with the fuel I'm using.

There are a lot of things that could potentially hinder adaptation, which I came to the conclusion of from my own experience. Before jumping in head first we need to keep in mind several important factors concerning keto and IF.

Too Many Carbs to Adapt

The biggest mistake we could make is to consume too many carbohydrates. Generally, they need to be restricted to less than 30-50 grams per day, without the fiber, for our body to enter ketosis.

The problem with most low carb diets is that they do not restrict their sugar intake enough for the body to completely convert over to fat burning. Even consuming slightly too much will keep us on the peripheral areas of keto adaptation. This is the worst place to be in because we will not be able to shift our metabolism into efficiently using ketones or get enough energy from glucose.

To get the most out of that amount we ought to be consuming only green leafy vegetables and not waste our allowance on things that don't satiate us as much.

Sugar hides itself in all shapes and form. Processed meat usually has added wheat or is cured in dextrose. Even though some foods might be keto friendly, such as heavy whipping cream, cheese and nuts, they still have a significant amount of sugar in them. That is why it's important to read the labels of everything that has one, as they can potentially spike our insulin. It almost resembles deciphering the complex linguistics of some ancient tablets because it can be quite complex.

How to Read Nutrition Labels

There are some national variations in terms of terminology, quantities and legislations but the core principles remain the same as long as we interpret the data according to our individual context. Put on your Indiana Jones' hat because this requires a lot of deciphering and linguistic work.

This is just a random example about what's most relevant and will guide you to making better decisions.

Here's a random label:

Nutrition Facts	
Serving Size 172 g	
Amount Per Serving	
Calories 200	Calories from Fat 8
	% Daily Value*
Total Fat 1g	1%
Saturated Fat 0g	1%
Trans Fat	
Cholesterol 0mg	0%
Sodium 7mg	0%
Total Carbohydrate 36g	12%
Dietary Fiber 11g	45%
Sugars 6g	
Protein 13g	
Vitamin A 1% • Vitamin C	1%
Calcium 4% • Iron	24%

*Percent Daily Values are based on a 2,000 calorie diet. Your daily values may be higher or lower depending on your calorie needs.

NutritionData.com

INGREDIENTS: ENRICHED FLOUR (WHEAT FLOUR, NIACIN, REDUCED IRON, THIAMIN MONONITRATE [VITAMIN B$_1$], RIBOFLAVIN [VITAMIN B$_2$], FOLIC ACID), CORN SYRUP, SUGAR, SOYBEAN AND PALM OIL (WITH TBHQ FOR FRESHNESS), CORN SYRUP SOLIDS, DEXTROSE, HIGH FRUCTOSE CORN SYRUP, FRUCTOSE, GLYCERIN, CONTAINS 2% OR LESS OF COCOA (PROCESSED WITH ALKALI), POLYDEXTROSE, MODIFIED CORN STARCH, SALT, DRIED CREAM, CALCIUM CARBONATE, CORNSTARCH, LEAVENING (BAKING SODA, SODIUM ACID PYROPHOSPHATE, MONOCALCIUM PHOSPHATE, CALCIUM SULFATE), DISTILLED MONOGLYCERIDES, HYDROGENATED PALM KERNEL OIL, SODIUM STEAROYL LACTYLATE, GELATIN, COLOR ADDED, SOY LECITHIN, DATEM, NATURAL AND ARTIFICIAL FLAVOR, VANILLA EXTRACT, CARNAUBA WAX, XANTHAN GUM, VITAMIN A PALMITATE, YELLOW #5 LAKE, RED #40 LAKE, CARAMEL COLOR, NIACINAMIDE, BLUE #2 LAKE, REDUCED IRON, YELLOW #6 LAKE, PYRIDOXINE HYDROCHLORIDE (VITAMIN B$_6$), RIBO-FLAVIN (VITAMIN B$_2$), THIAMIN HYDROCHLORIDE (VITAMIN B$_1$), CITRIC ACID, FOLIC ACID, RED #40, YELLOW #5, YELLOW #6, BLUE #2, BLUE #1.

1. The serving information. We'll start from the very top. This will tell you the size of a single serving and the total amount of them per package. These are random measurements not recommendations and the food companies can use them to trick uneducated readers.

2. **Calories per serving.** A bag of chips may have only 100 calories per serving, but the entire bag has 5 of them, totaling in 500 calories. This may trick you into believing that the entire small bag is one serving, whereas it has 5. I wouldn't bother making real interpretations based solely on calories per serving. The best way to understand this data is to calculate it to 100 grams instead.

3. **Macronutrient ratios.** Next, check out all of the macros. It's important to also see what proportions each of them contain. Be aware of the amount of trans fats and sugars. In the case of carbohydrates note how much of it is fiber as it may differ from the actual soluble content. I would completely ignore the % of daily values because the public recommendations are not individualized and taken out of context. It's based on an average 2000 calorie SAD diet and might be completely the opposite to what we need.

We only want to know the amounts we will be consuming and adjust that according to our own demands.

4. **Micronutrients.** The same applies to the vitamins. There is not much use to knowing how many micronutrients we're getting. If anything, then they're more likely put there to distract the reader away from all of the other potential hazards and bring in more confusion. Our individual deficiencies play a role here as well and we don't necessarily need everything. A much better way is to go to your doctor and get a blood test telling you exactly what vitamins you're deficient of.

5. **Ingredients.** They have to be listed in order of quantity with the major ones coming first. Some of them should also have exact percentages and amounts. All of the allergens or hazards are bolded for faster recognition but it varies between countries. Make sure you read and understand all of them and steer away from the dangers.

In the United States if a food has less than 0,5 grams of trans fat in a serving, the label can have 0 grams of it. This hidden sources will add up if you eat too much and can be the

314

hidden source of your problems. That's why it's important to also check the ingredient list for the actual contents for hydrogenated fats and vegetable oils.

Hidden Carbs

Additionally, what needs to be counted towards the daily carbohydrate allowance is seasoning. Industrialized mixes like lemon pepper or table salt are already contaminated with dextrose and, therefore, ought to be avoided like wildfire.

Natural spices, like cinnamon, turmeric and ginger also have a minute carbohydrate content, although most of it is fiber. We should be using them for their other medicinal benefits but be careful not to go overboard. This was one of the missing pieces of the puzzle that slowed down my adaptation the first time. I used to sprinkle seasoning on everything but didn't count them towards my daily carb allowance.

List of foods to avoid:

- All types of tubers, such as carrots, turnips, beetroot, potatoes.

- All grain products, such as rice, flour, wheat, barley, rye, quinoa.
- All legumes and lentils.
- All fruit, such as bananas, apples, oranges, grapes, watermelon etc.
- No yogurt with added sugar, no sodas, no milk, no chocolate, no cookies, no chips etc.

Too Much Protein

After eating too many carbohydrates, the next possible thing that hinders adaptation would be *gluconeogenesis*. Eating too much protein can convert even the juiciest of stakes into cake in our blood stream. What you don't need right away gets turned into sugar because during withdrawal every ounce of glucose is valuable. The body will sniff out whatever it can find.

However, for that to happen we would have to be consuming quite a lot. The recommended daily allowance for protein is already very low in comparison to what we would benefit from. How much we need depends on our weight and activity levels.

A sedentary person doesn't need nearly as much as someone who trains hard. If you're a small woman, then your requirements would be less than 100 grams per day. However, an athlete ought to be minimally consuming 0.8 grams per pound of lean body mass or 2 grams per kilogram, which is quite low and not nearly as much as the bodybuilding gurus tell us to eat.

The maximum we could get away with would be 1 g/pound. Anything higher than that will potentially turn into sugar. All kinds of whey powders and shakes are just another way to get money out of people by overemphasizing the importance of protein.

On the other hand, if you're doing a lot of resistance training *ala* Keto Bodybuilding (a must read for low carb strength trainees) and you're interested in packing on some lean muscle mass, then you would greatly benefit from a higher protein consumption. This doesn't mean that you should eat any more than 1.2-1.4 grams per pound of bodyweight because otherwise you'll overshoot IGF-1 and insulin. Eating too much protein when your body won't use it for building muscle will contribute towards tumor and cancer growth.

Ketosis is actually protein sparing because of the constant anabolic state we're in. Muscles will always have enough calories around and don't need to break down the body's own tissue and organs for energy.

After you've become fat adapted you don't have to worry about this as much. If you eat too much protein you'll get kicked out of ketosis, but only for a short period of time. Once a few hours have passed you'll re-enter the fat burning zone.

Not Enough Fat...What?

Another mistake would be not eating enough fat. As weird as it might sound that could happen. By eliminating carbohydrates from the menu we need to have another fuel source to feed our hungry brain. This means putting butter and olive oil over everything. The symptoms of withdrawal can be minimized by not adding caloric restriction on top of the adaptation process.

If we give our body more fat it will inevitably have to accept it. Moreover, this will also promote the liver's production of additional ketone bodies. On keto, you would rarely eat less than 150-200 grams of fat per day, unless you're very lightweight. What needs to be avoided, however, are the wrong types of fats, such as vegetable oils and trans fats, because of their inflammatory properties.

After all of the other macronutrients have been dialed in and potential infiltrations of sugar removed it's only a matter of time. It takes a lot of patience to get into ketosis. Quantifying with Ketostix or a glucometer would tell us about our progress but we shouldn't get caught up with the numbers. We can easily become consumed by it which would make things only worse.

Mistakes of IF

There are also a lot of common mistakes inexperienced practitioners could make when doing intermittent fasting. Here are a few guidelines to remember.

Don't Get Addicted to Coffee

Caffeine is an incredible appetite suppressant and reduces any hunger for many hours by increasing our focus and giving us energy. At the same time, it can also turn into a powerful drug.

A lot of people are like zombies when it comes to drinking coffee. They wake up, barely crawl out of bed and immediately reach out for a cup. What's worse, they add sugar and milk to it, making it even more stimulating. After the effects of wakefulness have diminished, they make another one and another one until they've become completely numb to it. It's a sad thing to see someone being addicted to anything, even something so seemingly innocent.

As in the case with insulin, the more we release it, the more resistant we become. You get used to running on caffeine and the added dose of sugar can make you feel like you can keep going. To maintain our sensitivity, we have to receive its stimulus less often.

While fasting we shouldn't drink more than 2-4 cups of coffee a day, nor should we feel the need to. When in mild ketosis, we'll already be having more energy and caffeine is just a nice thing to have.

I love coffee but I'm always mindful of how much and how often I'm consuming it. It's actually extremely good for us. If the beans are organic and free from mold, then the drink acts like an antioxidant. It also increases fat oxidation and sharpens our cognition. The famous philosopher of the Enlightenment

Voltaire used to drink more than 10 cups a day, but I wouldn't recommend you do that.

One of the best ways to maintain your sensitivity to caffeine is to cycle between regular coffee and decaf. They both taste the same and will suppress your appetite as much. To be honest, there isn't much difference in flavor. I tend to drink decaf for the majority of the week and use regular coffee whenever I feel like I need an extra boost. I'm not dependent of any stimulation and will thus remain *antifragile*.

For a full tutorial on how to drink coffee like a strategic mother#%a, read the Bonus Chapter.

Don't Get Dehydrated

We should instead increase our water intake. Drinking 8 cups of water a day isn't enough, especially while we're fasting.

Coffee is a diuretic and will increase dehydration. Compensate that with adding a bit of sea salt into your water. This will improve fluid absorption and keeps the electrolytes in balance.

Even just a few percentages of dehydration can lead to muscle cramps, exhaustion and decreased physical performance. You have to stay hydrated throughout the day. Gulping down 2 liters at once will only make you urinate it all out.

A cool little strategy to remind yourself to drink more is to use a huge water gallon and paint a hydration chart on it to keep track of your progress. Here's an example.

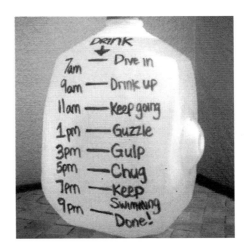

Although very effective and a great way to quantify your intake, you shouldn't become too reliant of it. Instead, get into the habit of carrying a water bottle with you and zipping on it every once in a while. You shouldn't feel obligated to drink if you're not thirsty or if you have to go to the bathroom too often.

The Untold Fight Club Rules of Intermittent Fasting

Intermittent fasting has a lot of unseen rules that no one talks about nor should. They're almost like agreed upon terms that resemble those in the movie Fight Club.

- ***The First Rule of Fight Club is: You do not talk about the Fight Club.***

Don't do fasting to become some sort of a martyr. The 19th century German philosopher Friedrich Nietzsche would agree with me on this: *"Wherever on earth the religious neurosis has appeared we find it tied to three dangerous dietary demands: solitude, fasting, and sexual abstinence. (Beyond Good and Evil : §47)"*

Fasting shouldn't be some sort of a means to *"repent our sins."* It's an empowering strategy that causes advantageous metabolic adaptations and hormonal responses, which we use to augment our body.

- ***The Second Rule of Fight Club is: You do not talk about the Fight Club!***

It's not a means of punishing oneself either. We shouldn't do intermittent fasting as restriction but instead as something that liberates and empowers us. Simply doing it in some shape or form is enough.

Restricting your eating window seems obsessive and confining but it actually gives you more freedom than ever before. You become less dependent of food and don't have to spend time eating just because you feel obligated to do so.

- *The Third Rule of Fight Club is: If someone yells "stop!", goes limp, or taps out, the fight is over.*

Doing intermittent fasting requires self-mastery, but it's also a double-edged sword. It asserts dominance over our unconscious urges but at the same time can be taken too far.

You need to be mindful about the conditions of your body and how well you can handle fasting. The fact is that physiologically you'll be fine. It's just that psychologically you may not be prepared for abstaining from food for long periods of time.

Don't jump into it right away if you can't handle it. Start with having 14 hour fasts, then 16, then 18 and then have your first 24-hour fast. If you want to go beyond that, then be my guest, but do so at your own risk and concern.

- *Fourth Rule: Only two guys to a fight.*

Don't try to impress someone else or get attached to an expected outcome. Fasting is a way to get more in tune with your own body and empower your body. It's you versus yourself, first and foremost.

You shouldn't force it onto others either. Everyone could use a bit of intermittent fasting but not all of them have the desire or the guts to eat only one meal a day. That's fine, you do your own thing. Those who want to follow the same path will have to choose to do so themselves.

- *Fifth Rule: One fight at a time, fellows.*

Fasting is a hormetic stressor to the body that needs to be taken in the right dose for it to have a positive response. The benefits will kick in only when the stimulus is just enough to force us to adapt but not too much for us to handle.

There's a fine line between anxiety and boredom; and anabolism and catabolism. It's a balancing act that requires a lot of attention and self-awareness.

If you're doing daily fasts of 20+ hours, then you should be mindful of other stressors you may come across. <u>Most common is probably training.</u> It's a lot stronger stimulus than fasting and when you add these two on top of each other you get a very powerful catabolic effect. In the right amounts it can be beneficial, however, in that case you would have to scale down either the intensity or frequency of your exercise. Doing this every single day without giving your body time to recover will over-stimulate your adrenals and lead to adrenal fatigue. That's when you've completely reached burnout and your organism is fighting for its life.

Additional stressors include lack of sleep and excessive exposure to artificial light at night. Blue light in the evening can offset our circadian rhythm and thus block the expression of some hormones.

Remember, most of the growth hormone gets released during the first few hours of sleep, at about 11-12PM. If you're on your gadgets at that time, then you may miss out on a lot. At least you won't be able to get into a deep state of repair by that time, as blue light will also stop the production of melatonin, the sleep hormone.

Sleep deprivation lowers testosterone and can cause insulin resistance. <u>Only a few hours of sleep for several nights in a row will make your blood sugar levels rise to that of a diabetic</u>. If you stay there for too long, you'll eventually get sick yourself. Don't think that you can get away with this, because eventually it will catch up with you.

Your body will only start to repair itself when its sleeping. All of the repair mechanisms and waste removal happens at night. That's also when we're building muscle and getting stronger. An adequate stimulus needs to be recovered from for full adaptation to occur.

- ***Sixth Rule: No shirts. No shoes.***

Another mistake would be to get too cold. It's a stress response like any other, as the body will always try to maintain its core temperature. Shivering is a way to produce endogenous heat and shows that your internal thermostat is working hard.

During fasting you may feel more cold than you normally would. If your fingers and toes are getting numb or blue, then you should stop and cover yourself up. Dress warmly and don't push yourself too hard.

- *Seventh Rule: Fights will go on as long as they have to.*

The positive effects of hormesis occur with just the right dosage. If you take it too far then you'll be actually causing more harm than good. Adaptations occur gradually and need to happen progressively.

At first your body won't be able to cope with fasting as well as it will later. Your fat burning ketogenic pathways have to be re-created before you can effectively utilize them.

Some signs of too much fasting are constant headaches, fatigue, feeling like being hit with a club, not sleeping well, shivering and feeling very cold despite wearing a lot of clothes. Be mindful of how your body reacts and listen to the signs that you're being given. Pushing it too far will lead to burnout and won't result with an advantageous outcome.

A word on gorging after fasting.

Intermittent fasting loses all of its beauty if you still eat like a scavenger all the time. It shouldn't be a means of eating more food, but a way to get away with eating less, without losing muscle and strength.

The Buddha also realized this, as he found that complete abstinence wasn't necessary. After he broke his 72 day fast, he started practicing moderation instead. That's the key idea we should take away here. When it comes to eating, walk the golden path in the middle. But also practice antifragility, which is by nature an extreme event.

- *And the Eight and Final Rule: If this is your first night at Fight Club, you have to fight.*

If you've made it this far in the book, then hopefully you've realized that intermittent fasting has a lot of benefits. It should also mean that you should incorporate it into your habitual eating plan. What's more, you should do it keto style.

Start restricting your feeding window to a certain degree and bring in regular fasts of 24+ hours. You don't have to make it too frequent but you should make it one of your annual fitness goals.

Watch the video about all of the rules on my YouTube channel.

My channel name is Siim Land (https://www.youtube.com/watch?v=rkz1ENQzt_k&t=13s).

Don't Eat Whatever

Intermittent fasting is a great way to create a caloric deficit. Because you'll be eating less often, your meals can be larger in quantities and calories. This can also mean that you're able to eat some junk food, while still maintaining a negative energy balance.

For *if it fits your macros* (IIFYM) type of flexible dieting it may work, but it's not optimal for overall health. Of course, the 80-20 rule can be applied here as well, and some indulgence here and there does you no harm.

At the same time, you should also consider what you're trying to accomplish with your nutrition in general. Is food just calories, or is it something more powerful? One thing is certain – eating causes certain metabolic adaptations and processes within the body. The hormonal response is a lot more important for longevity.

All in all, we should maintain this zen-like attitude towards the whole experience and simply let things everything run their course. Rather than being frustrated or lethargic we have to accept it as it is. We can't control what happens to us but only our response to it.

It ought to be something we enjoy and can later reflect back upon as an opportunity to learn more about our own body. Don't stress out on your ketone levels either. There isn't a specific point where we will become fat adapted but eventually we'll simply get accustomed to this new alteration of our own biology.

Chapter Takeaway:

- Don't eat more than 30-50 grams during the first few weeks of adaptation. Later you don't have to worry about it that much.
- Learn how to read nutrition labels properly and make sure all of the ingredients are safe to consume.
- Don't eat too much protein. This is easily solvable by swapping out lean bits with fatty chunks. Go full fat everything, expect in your adipose tissue. The maximum

you could consume is 0.8 to 1 gram per pound of lean body weight.

- Eat enough fat. Don't restrict your calories that much during adaptation.
- Don't get addicted to coffee. Use it strategically only when necessary and cycle off from it every few weeks.
- Don't be stressed out. Just chill and relax.
- Drink slightly more water than normally but don't overhydrate yourself. Look at your urine and frequency of going to the bathroom. Use added salts to keep your electrolytes in balance.
- Sleep at least 7-8 hours of sleep and try following the circadian rhythm. Get blue light blocking glasses and install Flux.
- Follow the Untold Fight Club Rules of Intermittent Fasting. Done.

Chapter Six

Recipes for Keto Fasting

You might think that what kind of a book about fasting has recipes? Of course, the strategies outlined here make us abstain from eating for a certain time frame but that is only so intermittently. We can't nor should fast indefinitely and that's why a you would want to include some feasting into the mix.

The amounts of any specific ingredient isn't important, unless it's in actual context. How much you ultimately eat is up to your own choosing. It varies between individuals and what they're trying to accomplish. However, we still want our first meal of the day to be relatively small so that we would remain slightly underfed.

Breakfast of Champions

What I mean by breakfast is the first meal of the day. The best "breakfast" we could ever have is a glass of water with salt in it and a healthy dose of intermittent fasting.

The minimum amount of fasting I would recommend for everyone is 14-16 hours. After you wake up, wait a few hours and don't rush into eating.

The most classical and satiating meal we could have are eggs and bacon. They have a lot of fat and protein with the right nutritional profile for high end performance. Additionally, we want some fiber and more fat. Even though I would recommend eating eggs for DHA and cholesterol it might not be possible because of allergies. The substitute for that or meat would be oily fish such as sardines, salmon, trout etc. The omega-3 fatty acids and EPA are even more beneficial for our cognition.

- **Ingredients**
  - 3 Eggs
  - 1 slice of bacon or 1 oz/28g of fish/sausage
  - 1oz/28g of spinach/collard greens/broccoli/cabbage
  - 1 tbsp butter/lard/ghee/coconut oil
  - Optional additives would be cheese or avocado.

- The spices would be pink Himalayan salt or regular sea salt, black pepper, turmeric, ginger, Cayenne pepper, cinnamon.

- **Preparation**
  - Either fry your eggs in a lot of butter, poach or boil them. Don't use too much heat as it will damage the nutrients. Throw in the bacon and mix the spinach in the same grease to coat it with fat.

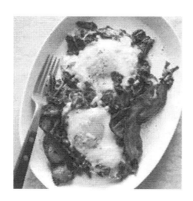

Approximate calories: 450-500 calories (35g protein/40g fat/2g carbs)

To wash it all down with we would also want something to drink. I'm going to share with you my secret recipe that will change your life forever.

Fatty Egg Yolk Coffee

The name of this recipe might be somewhat shocking. Don't worry, you'll change your opinion once you've tasted it. It's not entirely my own idea and I must say kudos to Dave Asprey the Bulletproof executive. However, my own version of it is even better. If you don't drink coffee, you can also use tea as a substitute.

- **Ingredients:**

  - Coffee/tea

  - 1 tbsp of butter/coconut oil/heavy cream/MCT oil

  - 1 whole egg

  - 1 tsp of raw cacao nibs, coconut flakes, Chaga mushroom, kelp powder and Chia seeds

  - 1/4 of an avocado seed, chopped. Yes, the avocado seed is very nutritious. You won't even notice the taste and will love the crunch it brings to your drink.

  - 1 tsp of cinnamon, turmeric, black pepper, sea salt and ginger

- **Preparation:**

  - o Brew your beverage and let it simmer for a while.

  - o Put the egg in your cup and break it down. If it stays in tact it will poach once you add the hot water.

  - o Throw in some cacao nibs, coconut flakes, chia seeds, about 5-10 grams each.

  - o Chaga mushroom and sea kelp powder, 1/2 teaspoon each because they're quite intense in flavor.

  - o Add 1 teaspoon of butter, coconut oil, heavy cream or MCT oil – which one you like most.

  - o Chop down the avocado seed into tiny parts with a knife and put them in the cup.

  - o Sprinkle in cinnamon, turmeric, ginger, black pepper and sea salt. You can also try out Cayenne pepper for an extra kick.

  - o Then mix it vigorously with a spoon or use a blender to create a nice froth on the surface. Using a blender will break the avocado seeds and other ingredients into an amazing mixture. Shaken not stirred, please.

o Take a sip and be amazed.

Approximate calories: 250 (10g protein/20g fat/2g carbs)

It looks very appealing and has some pools of grease on the surface. Taste it and be amazed as all of your taste buds will fire up. This beverage gives instant and long lasting energy for hours. You won't experience any crash that accompanies drinking coffee either because the fat slows down the release of caffeine. There won't be any quick spike or drop and the brain will function at its best. All of the neurons will light up with joy and are satisfied.

Bacon and Egg Muffins

If you like to eat breakfast then I'm not going to stop you from doing so. Whatever suits your condition. Maybe you like to cook in the morning and do nothing else. In that case, the following recipes are for the more serious keto chef.

- **Ingredients**
  o 2 tbsp of heavy cream

- 5oz/120g mushrooms, chopped
- 2 medium tomatoes, chopped
- 6 slices of bacon
- 4 eggs
- ¼ cup cheddar cheese, grated
- Seasoning according to preference

- **Preparation**

  - Preheat the oven to 375 degrees F (190 degrees C).
  - Cook the bacon strips on a frying pan on medium to low heat until crisp.
  - Use the bacon fat to grease the muffin cups.
  - Place one slice of bacon into each muffin cup so that the bacon lines the edges of the cup, like in a circle.
  - Beat the eggs and cream together, then pour them into muffin cups.
  - Bake in the oven until the muffins get slightly moist on top, which takes about 20 minutes. Season them with salt and pepper. Cover them with grated cheese and continue baking for about 5 minutes until melted.

- o Let the muffins cool down a bit and then remove them from the cups.
- o Enjoy small mouth-sized bites!

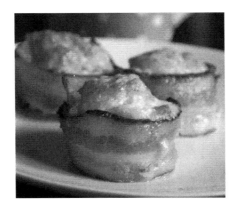

Approximate calories: 1000-1200 (90g protein/100g fat/2g carbs)

Approximate calories per muffin: 220 (15g protein/17g fat/0.5g carbs).

This recipe covered 6 muffins but you can change the quantities as much as you'd like. It's simple – 1 bacon strip for each cup.

Coconut Cream Porridge

It's thought that oatmeal is incredibly healthy. Well, it might be, but it's definitely not optimal because of gluten and the phytates found in whole grains.

Nevertheless, there's still a way to have a bowl of keto porridge that tastes equally as good and doesn't come with any negative effects.

- **Ingredients**
  - o 1 cup of coconut cream
  - o 1 oz of almonds (about 20), ground or whole
  - o 1 teaspoon of cinnamon and Stevia (optional)
  - o 1 teaspoon of coconut flakes
  - o A pinch of nutmeg
- **Preparation**
  - o Heat the coconut cream on a saucepan on medium until it forms a liquid.
  - o Add the almonds, coconut flakes and stevia
  - o Mix well and keep stirring for a few minutes until it begins to thicken.
  - o Add the cinnamon, nutmeg and taste.

o Serve hot.

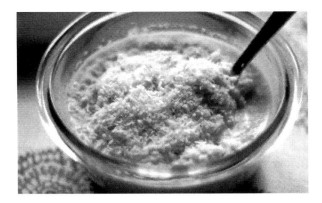

Approximate calories: 750 calories (15g protein/70g fat/15g carbs)

After having a delicious and satiating breakfast, you shouldn't get hungry at all until the evening. If you do, simply add some more fat to your meals. Eating less frequently is the ideal worth striving towards. Two times a day is the golden mean.

Moving on with some amazing dinner recipes you can use to treat your entire family in the evening with or host a party with your friends.

Keto Pizza Frittata

Here's an amazing *Italian-esque* dish that's even tastier than the regular pizza. This entire batch should have about 4 servings.

- **Ingredients**
  - 1 teaspoon sea salt, fennel seeds, onion powder, ground sage, pepper, dried parsley
  - 2 oz/50g of ground pork
  - 5 eggs
  - 2 cups of tomatoes cooked into a sauce
  - 2 oz/50 g cheese
  - 1 tablespoon coconut oil or butter
  - 1 bell pepper, sliced
  - 1 cup of mushrooms, sliced
  - 2 cup sliced onions
  - 2-4 scallions, sliced
- **Preparation**
  - Preheat the oven to 400F/200C.
  - Heat a large skillet over medium heat.
  - Combine the ground pork and spices in a mixing bowl.

o Add the meat to the skillet and cook for about 10 minutes until only slightly pink is left. After this set aside the pan for now.

o Whisk together the eggs, add salt and pepper.

o Stir together the tomato sauce, add seasoning.

o Melt the coconut oil over medium heat and cook the bell pepper until it starts to soften, for about 5 minutes.

o Add the mushrooms later and cook for about 2 minutes.

o Put back the meat and add scallions. Mix and combine all of the ingredients.

o Pour in the egg mixture and tile the pan around until they cover the entire bottom.

o Let the frittata to cook for about 5 minutes until it starts to get slightly soft on the edges.

o Drizzle the tomato sauce over the mixture, sprinkle the cheese on top, then put the pan in the oven for 8-10 minutes. To check if done, use a knife to cut into the mix. If still runny, cook for another few minutes.

- Before serving, let it cook for about 5 minutes and then cut into pieces.

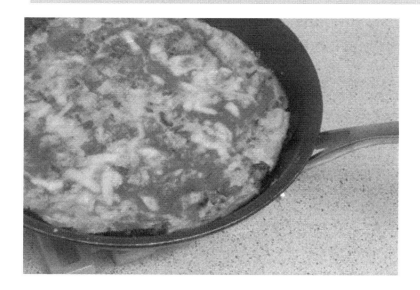

Approximate calories for the entire batch: 900(70g protein/60g fat/6g carbs).

Approximate calories per ¼ of the frittata: 250 (20g protein/15g fat/2g carbs).

Perfect Roasted Chicken

Cook an entire chicken - enough said.

- **Ingredients**
  - 1 whole chicken

- Salt and pepper
- 1 bunch of fresh thyme and rosemary
- 1 lemon cut in half
- 1 head of garlic
- 2 tablespoons of extra virgin olive oil
- 1 medium onion cut in quarters

- **Preparation**

  - Preheat the oven to 400 F /200 C.
  - You can cut the thighs and wings into separate pieces or simply put the entire chicken onto a pan.
  - Make a dissection into the chicken and sprinkle in some salt and pepper inside.
  - Stuff the cavity with thyme, lemon and garlic. Add some sea salt on top of the skin to let it melt in.
  - Tie the legs together and tuck the wings under the body.
  - Place the onion quarters at the corners of the dish.
  - Cook the chicken for about an hour or until juices run clear.
  - 5 minutes before finishing, brush the chicken with olive oil.

o Before eating, allow it to slightly cool.

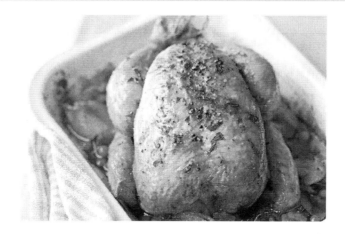

Approximate calories with 1 pound of chicken: 1000(80g protein/80g fat/1g carb from the lemon).

Meaty Vegetable Roast Feast

This is one of the best staple dinners we could ever have. It's quick and super easy to make with little to no effort involved. The actual ingredients aren't as important as we can use anything. What matters are only the amounts and the idea.

- **Ingredients:**
  - o Some source of fatty meat. Beef, pork chops, chicken wings, thighs etc.

- Some source of leafy green vegetables. Cabbage, cauliflower, spinach, broccoli, collard greens etc.
- Some source of extra fat. Butter, lard, ghee, olive oil etc.
- Spices according to your liking.

- **Preparation:**
  - Grab a pan and add all of the ingredients by placing the greens on the bottom and the meat on top. Sprinkle bits of coarse sea salt on the meat so it would melt into it. Additionally, you can squeeze some lemon juice as well. Pour a bit of water into the bottom. Don't add any extra fat yet.
  - Put it all in the oven and let it cook for about 30-45 minutes. As its starting to be finished throw some butter on top. Don't heat olive oil because it will oxidize and cause inflammation. Use it afterwards as dressing instead.
  - Mix all of the vegetables inside the fat. As a sider you can add some avocados or nuts. Dinner is served.

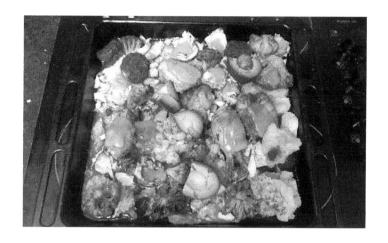

Approximate calories for 1 pound of dish: 750(50g protein/60g fat/6g carbs).

Cauliflower Pizza.

The most amazing and versatile food at our disposal on keto is cauliflower. It can be used to substitute almost anything we're used to having: mashed potatoes, rice and pizza. This recipe will teach you how to have your gluten-free-low-carb crust that fits ketosis perfectly.

- **Ingredients:**

  - 1 head of Cauliflower

  - 2-3 Eggs

- 1 cup of Tomatoes

- ½ cup of Cheese

- 1 oz/25g of olives

- Seasoning and herbs of your choosing.

- **Preparation:**

  - Take the entire head of a cauliflower and cut off the florets.

  - In a food processor shred them all into bits and pieces.

  - Add in an egg or two and blend the mixture.

  - Spread the mixture on a pan and put it in the oven for 30 minutes at 375 F/190 C.

  - This will turn into a crust and creates texture.

  - Add the tomatoes and cheese on top and let it cook for a while until ready.

The same can be done with zucchini as well. Instead of it being pizza they look like boats instead. Simply cut the vegetable in half and add the other ingredients. Cook it in the oven until the cheese starts to melt down and you'll have a quick meal.

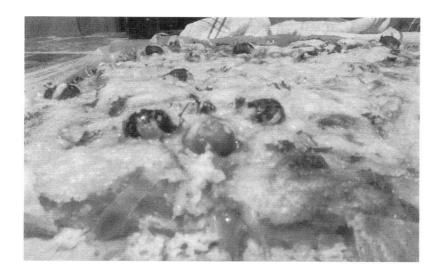

Approximate calories for the entire pizza: 900 (50g protein/40g fat/20g carbs).

Approximate calories for ¼ of the pizza: 250(15g protein/10g fat/5g carbs).

Bone Broth Soup

We've been referring back to the importance and benefits of this recipe, so here it is.

One of the biggest downsides to eating keto is that some mineral deficiencies might occur. That isn't caused by the lack of variety in the diet but by the low nutritional quality of our soils and vegetables.

To circumvent that we would have to take some supplements. However, there is another way. It's even better and a great way to get in touch with our primal side.

When a hunter-gatherer caught an animal nothing was wasted. Meat was a precious source of calories and they ate everything that was edible. Instead of trimming off the fat they went for the good stuff. Liver, kidneys, heart, bone marrow, skin with fat on – those are the most nutritious parts. It's only in today's contemporary society where people get disgusted by them.

Culture depicts organ meat as putrid and the lean bits as something pure whereas we would be better off by neglecting none. This recipe transcends this dichotomy between the wild and domesticated by incorporating an ancestral practice into our menu.

- **Ingredients:**

- Bones of a grass-fed and organically raised animal (chicken drumsticks, beef collar, wild boar bones etc.). Healthy animals will have stronger skeletomuscular structure.
- Onions, garlic.
- Optionally some organ meats such as: heart, kidneys, liver, chicken gizzards etc.
- Spices: laurel-leafs, unground pepper and coarse sea salt.

- **Preparation:**
  - Grab a big pot of water and throw in the ingredients. In order to get all of the minerals from the bones they need to be boiled for several hours on low heat. The longer they do the better. Put it on the stove at the beginning of the day and just let it sit there.
  - Add the organ meats only during the last hour of preparation as they would simply turn to pudding.
  - After a while the bones will begin to break down. Joints and tendons are the best because they have a lot of connective tissue attached to them. That's what we're after – the ligaments and the marrow inside.

Once that happens the water will turn into a pool of fat and grease which tastes amazing.

o Drops of liquid begin to float the surface and give the soup its flavor. It can be used as a basis for other types of cooking or simply drank as a beverage.

o Storing it is easy as it will turn gelatinous after cooling down which can then be re-heated afterwards.

The bone broth soup is a great way to get in all of the essential minerals and nutrients we need from animals. Not only is it tasty and heart-warming but also very good for the gut. It reduces overall inflammation and promotes the strength of our joints because of the marrow.

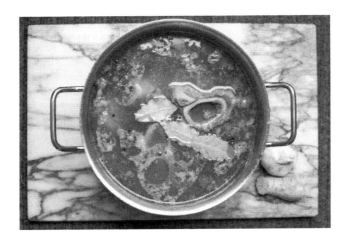

Approximate calories per 1 cup of soup: 110(5g protein/10g fat/0g carbs).

Now, after dinner you might also want something for dessert. Even though, you'll most likely lose your sweet tooth after keto adaptation, you can still enjoy treats that will light up your taste buds and bring you incredible satiation.

The ketogenic diet doesn't have any carbohydrates or sugar in the menu. Mostly, there's only bacon fat, butter and vegetables – not anything sweet. However, thinking that there aren't any desserts is a myth.

Almond Butter Fat Bombs

To get in enough calories from fat, you would have to use it liberally. The old days of using oils and butter sparingly are over. For this purpose, there are several *"fat-bomb"* recipes we can use to boost our lipid intake, without increasing our waistline. This recipe should make for about 5-7 fat bombs.

- **Ingredients**
  - 1/2 cups of almond butter
  - 1 tablespoon of coconut oil or butter

- 2 to 3 teaspoons of <u>Stevia</u> (optional)
- 2 teaspoons of <u>cacao nibs</u>
- 1 teaspoon of cinnamon
- 1 tablespoon of <u>coconut flakes</u>

- **Preparation**
  - Place all the ingredients in a pot and heat on medium heat for about 1 minute. Let the fat melt down slightly, but don't make it too liquid.
  - Whisk together the ingredients and pour the mixture into ice cube trays. Freeze for 2 hours.
  - Take the fat bombs out of the freezer and pop them out of the tray.
  - Either eat them right away or store them in the freezer for future use.
  - Enjoy your little bite-sized fat bombs.

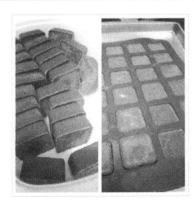

Approximate calories for the entire batch: 850 (20g protein/80g fat/5g carbs).

Approximate calories for 1 fat bomb: 130 (4g protein/12g fat/1g carbs).

Coconut Milk Ice Cream

Despite the lack of sugar in the diet it doesn't mean that we can't be having something sweet. To be honest, the umami taste of bacon feels like candy. Maybe it's just me. We can still have ice cream and bake cakes using keto friendly ingredients and they're even better. This recipe is completely dairy free and suitable for everyone.

- **Ingredients:**

    o 2 cups of coconut milk

    o 2 eggs

    o 2 tablespoons of butter and olive oil

    o 1 teaspoon of vanilla extract or Stevia (optional)

    o Nuts according to preference.

- o 1 tablespoon of coconut flakes

- o ½ cups of blueberries

- o 1 teaspoon of cinnamon

- **Preparation:**

  - o Separate the egg yolks and whites.

  - o Whip the whites until they turn soft.

  - o Mix vigorously or blend together butter, olive oil, seasoning while simultaneously adding in the yolks. Do it one by one and slowly until a smooth mixture forms.

  - o Pour in the coconut milk and slowly add the egg whites.

  - o Keep mixing it all together to make it more fluffy.

  - o It should begin to become thicker after a while. For texture add more eggs.

  - o Throw in the nuts, blueberries, coconut flakes and cinnamon.

- You can put it in the freezer for a few hours for it to turn more solid or eat right away. The perfect dessert for a hot day.

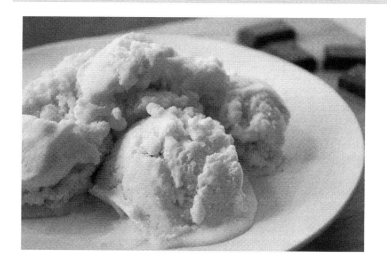

Approximate calories: 500 (20g protein/40g fat/5g carbs).

Keto Pancakes

Everyone's childhood is probably filled with memories about having pancakes on Sunday. They're great but not for our health because of the gluten and high-fat-carb combo. Fortunately, there is another solution – the keto way. By replacing some of the ingredients, we can still enjoy a healthy tasty dessert.

- **Ingredients:**

  - 2-3 eggs

  - 2 cups of coconut milk or heavy cream (has twice the calories)

  - 2 tablespoons of butter or coconut oil

  - 2oz/50g of almond or coconut flour

  - 1 teaspoon of cinnamon

  - 1/3 cup of blueberries and coconut flakes

- **Preparation:**

  - Beat the eggs until soft.

  - Pour in cream and flour according to preference and texture.

  - Mix them together with cinnamon.

  - Heat the pan with butter.

  - Pour in the pancake mixture and cook on both sides.

- While in the pan throw some coconut flakes on top.

- Serve on a plate with blueberries.

This recipe doesn't even have to involve flour. We can get the same results by using only eggs and cream. It won't look like batter but there hardly is any other difference.

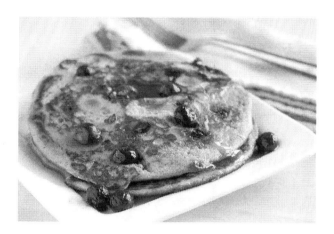

Approximate calories for 3 pancakes: 650 (40g protein/50g fat/6g carbs).

Keto Chocolate

You can eat dark chocolate on keto and it's incredibly healthy for your health. What's more, it tastes a lot better than the regular milk chocolate equivalent.

You can put only 1 small piece of 80%+ chocolate that's darker than night in your mouth and be incredibly satiated. Your taste buds will light up but won't cause any additional cravings.

Good quality dark chocolate can be hard to come by. No worries, you can make your own with.

- **Ingredients**
  - 2 tablespoons of coconut oil
  - 2 tablespoons of raw cacao butter
  - 3 tablespoons of cacao powder
  - 1 cup of coconut milk or almond milk (optional, if you want a milkier texture)
  - 1 teaspoon of vanilla extract
  - 1 teaspoon of cinnamon
  - A pinch of sea salt
  - 1 teaspoon of Stevia
- **Preparation**
  - Melt the coconut oil and cacao butter in a skillet over very low heat. Let the texture get softer slowly. Don't make it boil.
  - Once the mixture is melted, turn off the heat and mix in the cacao powder. It should look dark and creamy.

- If you want more of a milky taste, mix in the coconut milk.
- Stir in the cinnamon, salt, stevia and the vanilla extract.
- Allow the chocolate mixture to cool until it reaches room temperature.
- Put the mixture in the refrigerator for 30 minutes until it becomes solid.
- After the chocolate has solidified, break it apart and put it in a glass container.
- Savor the taste by eating small pieces at a time.

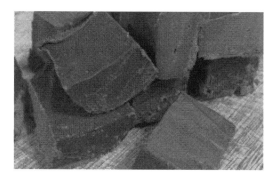

Approximate calories for the entire batch: 500 (5g protein/45g carbs/3g carbs).

Chapter Takeaway

- Although the ketogenic diet has a lot of limitations in terms of macronutrient ratios, there's still a lot of variety in the menu. You just have to use your creativity and imagination.
- There are amazing keto dishes you can make for breakfast, lunch and dinner that are all healthy, anti-inflammatory and satiating.
- You can use keto-friendly ingredients to cook almost all of your favourite food, such as pizza, ice cream, pancakes and chocolate. It takes just a little bit of extra effort and knowledge.

Chapter Seven

A Chapter About Supplementation

Despite our access to abundant contemporary food we're still missing some key ingredients - the micronutrients. To overcome this flaw there are some supplements we should be taking.

With the industrialization of food all of that has suffered. Our soils are being depleted from their vital life force with the use of fertilizers, spraying of toxic fumes, usage of GMOs, radiation, travel pollution and many other things. All for the purpose of creating more empty calories and food without any actually beneficial content.

A Word of Caution

There are a lot of supplements we could be taking. However, that doesn't mean we should start gorging on piles of tablets and numerous pills. It's not about becoming a substance junkie, but a self-empowered being who simply covers all of the necessary micronutrients through the usage of natural yet still manufactured additives.

We don't need to take a whole lot, simply some which everyone needs and especially those that we're individually most deficient of. That's something we have to find out ourselves.

All of the supplements that I have listed here are least processed and free from any additional garbage, such as preservatives, GMO, gluten, starch, sugar etc. They're keto-proof and friendly.

Additionally, we should always try to stick to real whole foods as much as possible. Supplements are just that - supplementation for some of the deficiencies we fail to get from what we actually eat. They're not magical but simply give us the extra edge.

The effects these products have can be derived from natural foods as well. In the form of a pill or a powder they're simply microscopic and packaged nutrition. Taking them will grant us access to optimal health - the utmost level of wellbeing and performance both physical and mental.

In this list are all of the supplements I am personally taking because of their importance, as well as the additional benefits we get. However, I do not advise anyone to take any of them unless they are aware of their medical condition and don't know about the possible side effects or issues that may or may not follow.

Before taking anything we ought to educate ourselves about the topic and consult a professional physician. <u>The responsibility is solely on the individual and I will take none.</u>

Natural Seasoning

To start off I'm going to list the supplements we should be taking, each and every one of us, as they are something that we're definitely all deficient of and also promote Superhuman wellbeing.

Not everything we consume ought to come in the form of a pill. A lot of micronutrients can be found in unprocessed products as well, we simply need to add them to our diet and reap the benefits. They are most natural and completely free from the touch of man. Therefore, they come first and are of utmost value.

We've already covered the health and medicinal properties of turmeric, ginger and cinnamon but in case you forgot, here they are again. You should start adding them to your food no matter what.

- **Turmeric.** One of the best spices we can use is curcumin or turmeric. It has a lot of medicinal properties, such as anti-inflammatory compounds, increase of antioxidants and brain health. Also, it fights and prevents many diseases, such as Arthritis, Alzheimer's and even cancer. In addition to that, it tastes amazing and can be added to everything. I sprinkle it on all foods and run out quite quickly which is why I also buy it in bulk so that it's cheaper. You can also take a capsule.

- **Ginger.** Continuing on with turmeric's brother. It has almost as much health benefits. In addition to that, it lowers blood sugar levels, fights heart disease, treats chronic indigestion, may reduce menstrual pain for women, lowers cholesterol and heals muscle pain. Once again, bulk or capsule.

- **Cinnamon.** These three create the most important natural spices we should be eating on a daily basis. They're incredibly cheap and easy to come by yet have amazing health as well as performance enhancing benefits. Moreover, they all make food taste amazing. Cinnamon falls into the same category as ginger and turmeric - superfoods, because it truly empowers us. In addition to the same medicinal properties it also increases insulin sensitivity, fights neurodegenerative disease and bacterial infections. What's best about it is that it can be added to not only salty foods but on desserts as well. I even add it to my coffee. The best to use is Ceylon or „true" cinnamon.

- **Green tea.** It isn't an actual supplement but is still extremely empowering. In fact, it can be considered to be the healthiest beverage of the world after water. It improves health, brain function, fat oxidation and detoxifies the system. Additionally, lowers blood pressure and prevents all types of disease, including Alzheimer's and cancer. We don't need to take pills with extracts but can get all of the benefits by simply drinking a cup a day.

However, to get all of the benefits we need to be consuming about 15-30 cups. Using a capsule would be very efficient.

- **Garlic.** It has a strong taste and smell but is incredibly healthy nonetheless. Chopping garlic cloves forms a compound called '*allicin*,' which, once digested, travels all over the body and exerts its potent biological effects. It fights all illness, especially the cold, reduces blood pressure, improves cholesterol levels, contains antioxidants, increases longevity, detoxifies the body from metals, promotes bone health and is delicious. Because of its flavor it makes a great addition to meals. It also comes in capsuled form.

Supplements you HAVE to Take

Moving on with actual supplements. These things we're all deficient of and they also take our performance to the next level, they empower us.

- **Fish/Krill oil.** It's rich in omega-3 fatty acids, which are great for the brain and heart. The counterpart to that is omega-6, which are pro-inflammatory and bad for us. Omega-6 can be found in a lot of processed foods and vegetable oils, which we would want to avoid anyway. For our body to be healthy the omega-3's need to be in balance with the omega-6's. Unfortunately, that balance can be easily tipped off as every amount of omega-6 requires triple the amount of omega-3 to reduce the negative effects. Additionally, fish oil has DHA, which promotes brain functioning, fights inflammation, supports bone health, increases physical performance etc. Naturally, it can be found in fatty fish such as salmon, herring, mackerel and sardines. Fish oil falls into the same category because of its vital importance for superhuman health. It can be used easily as a capsule or liquidized. Taking one teaspoon a day will drastically improve your life. Krill oil might simply be a more potent and bioavailable source. Make sure to use wild caught sources to avoid mercury poisoning.

- **Vitamin D-3.** It's called the sunshine vitamin and is one of the most important nutrients. But it's not actually a vitamin but gets synthesized into one inside the body. Life exists on Earth because of the Sun. D-3 governs almost every function within us starting from DNA repair and metabolic processes making it a foundation to everything that goes on. It's embedded in nutritious food, given it has received enough exposure to solar light. Vitamin D-3 fights cardiovascular, autoimmune and infective diseases. Of course, the best source would be to get it from the Sun but that is not always possible because of seasonality and location. It can be consumed as oil or a capsule.

- **Magnesium.** Another foundational mineral. It comprises 99% of the body's mineral content and governs almost all of the processes. Magnesium helps to build bones, enables nerves to function and is essential for the production of energy from food. This is especially beneficial for the physically active. Some people who are depressed get headaches because of this deficiency. Because our soils are quite depleted magnesium needs to be supplemented. It can also be used as an oil on your skin for greater absorption in specific areas.

Supplements Empowered

We have covered all of the supplements we should be taking no matter what, the most important and essential ones. Now I'll get down to the empowering ones.

They are not foundational but beneficial nonetheless. With the help of these we can transcend the boundary between healthy and superhuman performance as they will take us to the next level.

- **Creatine Monohydrate.** Creatine is an organic acid produced in the liver that helps to supply energy to cells all over the body, especially muscles. It enhances ATP production and allows for muscle fibers to contract faster, quicker, and makes them overall stronger. That means increased physical performance with explosive and strength based movements and sprinting. However, it doesn't end there. Creatine has been found to improve cognitive functioning, as it's a nootropic as well, improving mental acuity and memory. Naturally, it can be found most in red meat. It's dirty cheap and easy to consume, as only 5 grams per day will do wonders and doing so won't make a person big nor bulky.

- **Pro- and prebiotics.** Having a well working digestive system is incredibly vital for getting the most nutrients out of our food. Industrialization has done another disservice to us by destroying all of the bacteria in the food we consume, the good and the bad, and replacing them with preservatives. We might be eating but we're not actually deriving a lot of nutrients. In order to have a healthy gut we need to have a well-functioning microbiome. Naturally, food is full of living organisms. Sauerkraut, raw milk, yoghurt, unprocessed meat all have good bacteria in them. With there being no life in our food, we need to create it within us ourselves. Probiotics are alive microorganisms in a pill that transport these good bacteria into our gut for improved digestion and immune system. Prebiotics are different, they're not alive, but plant fiber that feeds the bacteria. They're indigestible parts of the vegetable that go through our digestive track into our gut where the bacteria then eat them. If you don't like eating a lot of broccoli and spinach, then you should still get a lot of fiber into your diet.

- **Thyroid supplementation.** The thyroid gland is incredibly important for our health because it regulates the functioning of our metabolism. Moreover, because of its location in our throat it also is a connective point between the brain and the rest of the body. This organ is a part of an incredibly complex system which creates this intertwined relationship between the two. With a low functioning thyroid one will have an impeded metabolism, suffer hypothyroidism and many other diseases because of the necessary hormones will not be produced. Promoting thyroid functioning can be done by taking iodine supplementation or eating a lot of sea vegetables. The daily requirements for selenium can be met with eating only 2-3 Brazil nuts.

- **Multivitamin.** There are definitely a lot of vitamins to be covered for our body to not only be healthy but function at its peak. It would be unreasonable to take too many tablets or pills while neglecting the importance of real food. However, taking a multivitamin that has a lot of beneficial minerals all combined into one bottle is very effective and will most definitely be useful.

- **Maca.** Another superfood comes from the Peruvian mountains and is the root of ginseng. It has numerous amounts of vitamins and minerals in it, such as magnesium zinc, copper etc. Also, it promotes hormone functioning for both men and women, as well as increases our energy production just like creatine does. It can either be powdered or made into a tablet.

- **GABA.** Called gamma-aminobutyric acid, it's the main inhibitory neurotransmitter, and regulates the nerve impulses in the human body. Therefore, it is important for both physical and mental performance, as both of them are connected to the nervous system. Also, GABA is to an extent responsible for causing relaxation and calmness, helping to produce BDNF.

- **Chaga mushroom.** Chaga is a mushroom that grows on birch trees. It's extremely beneficial for supporting the immune system, has anti-oxidative and soothing properties, lowers blood pressure and cholesterol. Also, consuming it will promote the health and integrity of the adrenal glands. This powder can be added to teas or other warm beverages. Or you can grind it yourself.

- **MCT oil.** For nutritional ketosis having an additional source of ketone bodies will be beneficial. MCT stands for medium chain triglycerides which are fat molecules that can be digested more rapidly than normal fat ones, which are usually long chain triglycerides. Doing so will enable the brain to have immediate access to abundant energy and a deeper state of ketosis. Basically, it's glucose riding the vessel of ketones. Naturally, it's extracted from coconut oil and is an enhanced liquidized version of it. Additionally, I also eat raw coconut flakes, which have MCTs in them.

- **Collagen protein.** Collagen provides the fastest possible healthy tissue repair, bone renewal and recovery after exercise. It can also boost mental clarity, reduce inflammation, clear your skin, promote joint integrity, reduces aging and builds muscle. Naturally, it's found in tendons and ligaments, that can be consumed by eating meat. As a supplement it can be used as protein powder or as gelatin capsules.

- **Branched Chain Amino Acids.** L-Leucine, L-Isoleucine, and L-Valine are grouped together and called BCAAs because of their unique chemical structure. They're essential and have to be derived from diet. Supplementing them will increase performance, muscle recovery and protein synthesis. There is no solid evidence to show any significant benefit to BCAAs. However, they can be very useful to take before fasted workouts to reduce muscle catabolism.

This is the list of supplements we should be taking. It includes the most important ones, the essential, which we should be taking no matter what, as well as the not so vital that simply make us more empowered and give us the extra edge. Nothing replaces good food, but proper and educated supplementation will fix some of the loopholes.

Chapter Takeaway

- Contemporary food doesn't have a lot of micronutrients in it because of poor soils, travel pollution and preservation.
- You have to take full responsibility over taking supplements. If you screw up something then you're the one to blame, not me.
- Natural seasoning, such as turmeric, ginger, cinnamon and garlic, make food taste amazing and promote superhuman health.
- You should definitely supplement omega-3s, magnesium and vitamin D-3.
- Use other empowering supplements according to your preference, goals and needs.

Bonus Chapter

How to Drink Coffee Like a Strategic MotherF#%ka!

One of the most commonly used performance enhancing drugs in the world – coffee. It's used by many vocations and has been fueling the progress of the Western society. Because of that, it also has its side-effects that can doom those who misuse this beverage.

Why Do People Drink Coffee?

Besides the great taste, it also has a ton of benefits to it. Long-term consumption of caffeine in the form of coffee is associated with cognitive enhancements[lxxv],reduced risk for type-2 diabetes[lxxvi], Alzheimer's[lxxvii] and Parkinson's[lxxviii].

Caffeine travels to the brain and blocks a neurotransmitter called Adenosine. As a result, <u>norepinephrine and dopamine actually increase, which hastens the firing rate of neurons</u>[lxxix].

Normal

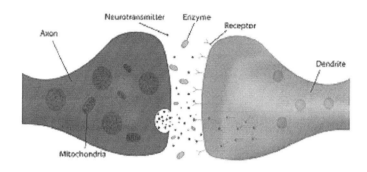

With Caffeine

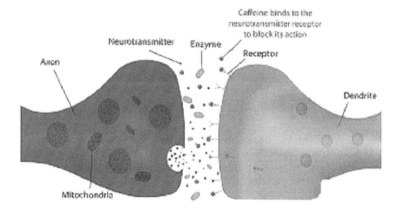

Drinking coffee is probably one of the most widespread brain power enhancers used by scientists and other vocations, such as writers or doctors, that demand a lot of cognitive output for long periods of time.

Coffee beans have a lot of antioxidants, called *quinines*, that fight disease and clean the body. After the roasting process, they become even more potent. They also contain naturally a lot of magnesium.

Is Coffee Bad for You?

What about the costs? Are there any negative side-effects?

You've probably seen people who have become addicted to coffee. It's a dreadful sight – their hands are jittering and they have anxiety. The reason is that they have simply taken advantage of caffeine the wrong way.

For the wide majority of people, it's safe. However, additional side-effects can be insomnia, upset stomach, increased heart rate and blood pressure.

In my opinion, **caffeine should be used only in certain situations when you actually need a boost.** It's just that – a performance enhancing stimulant that gives us the right amount of energy for whatever the task might be.

There's a much healthier way to drink coffee effectively, which I'm about to share with you, that circumvents most of those issues.

The Best Time to Drink Coffee

For the ordinary person, drinking coffee immediately after waking up is the only thing that gets them going. They open their eyes, roll out of the bed and have to crawl to get their dose of java ASAP. But those are first signs of dependence and overdosing.

It's not the ideal time to be consuming caffeine either. Coffee acts as a stimulant for the body that triggers some physiological processes. Our biology is already connected with the planetary movements and circadian rhythms.

Between the hours of 8-9 AM, our cortisol levels are at their peak[lxxx]. It's the *"fight or flight"* hormone, that rises in the morning so that we would have increased alertness and focus. We're already supposed to be fully alert and energized after waking up. So, if we simultaneously drink coffee, we're wasting the potential benefits of caffeine and offsetting the circadian rhythm.

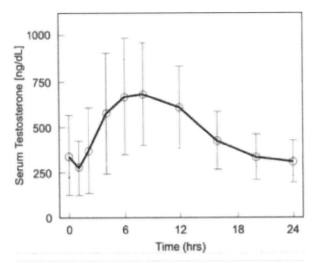

Figure 1. Diurnal variation of serum testosterone levels each day. The levels are highest in the early morning, dropping progressively during the day.

The best time to drink coffee is between 9:30 AM and 11:30 AM. Cortisol peaks in the early morning, but also fluctuates during the day. Other times it rises are 12 PM – 1 PM and 5:30 PM and 6:30 PM, so avoid a cup of joe at those hours as well.

When we're doing intermittent fasting, timing our coffee is even more relevant. If we were to cash in on one of our back-up cards, we would be left unarmed when hunger strikes.

Instead of drinking coffee immediately after we get hungry, we should first drink some water, then wait for about 30 minutes and only then decide whether or not it's worth it to have a nice cup of joe. In general, wait for a few hours after waking up before getting yours.

Drink Coffee - Can't Sleep

Drinking coffee at the wrong time can also keep you up and prevents you from falling asleep completely. You won't be able to get a good night's sleep and because of that wake up groggy and tired, you immediately grab another cup and the perpetual cycle continues.

The half-life of caffeine is about 5.7 hours[lxxxi], which means that if you drink coffee at 12 PM, then 50% of it will still be in your system at 6 PM. According to the circadian rhythm, the best time to go to bed is at about 9-11 PM. You should be sound asleep before midnight, because that's when the most growth hormone gets released.

Ingesting caffeine in the evening will definitely keep you up at night. <u>That's why you should stop drinking coffee after 2-4 PM in the afternoon.</u>

Are You a Fast Oxidizer or a Slow One

But some people don't report these issues. They can drink coffee even just a few hours before going to bed and still fall asleep just fine. What gives?

Our metabolism differs between individuals and we have our own unique type, which makes us metabolize nutrients at different speeds.

- **The fast oxidizer is someone who digests food very quickly and converts it into energy rapidly.** They need to focus on eating heavier meals with more fat and protein that would keep them satiated. By the same token, they will also absorb caffeine that much faster and it will go through their system almost at an instant.

- **If you're a slow oxidizer, then you need more time to convert food into energy.** Because of that, you require more carbohydrates, rather than protein and fat. Getting the benefits of coffee will also be less rapid.

How Much Coffee Should You Drink

An average cup of coffee contains 100-150 mg of caffeine, but you won't get the full benefits from just one cup.

Consuming caffeine in small but frequent amounts is more advantageous. The optimal dose for cognitive functioning may be 20-200 mg per hour[lxxxii].

Small hourly doses can support extended wakefulness, by acting against the homeostatic sleep pressure, which builds up slowly throughout the day[lxxxiii] and benefits the prefrontal cortex, which is responsible for higher executive functions[lxxxiv].

Doses of 600 mg are often comparable to the effects of modafinil, which is a top notch nootropic and cognitive enhancer. It's a smart drug but there are no reported advantages over large amounts of caffeine.

Various Doses of Caffeine

- For headaches or boosting alertness: 250 mg, or 2 cups per day.

- For preventing Parkinson's: 3 to 4 cups.

- For preventing type-2 diabetes: 900 mg, or 6 cups.

To avoid any unwanted side-effects, use filtered coffee. Darker roasts have less caffeine in them, due to the roasting process.

What Tasks Benefit the Most from Coffee

Drinking coffee won't make you a bad person, quite the opposite. There are also a lot of mood enhancing benefits that will make you more enjoyable to be around. Napoleon Bonaparte said: *"The only good thing about St Helena is the coffee."*

The famous French philosopher of the Enlightenment Voltaire was said to be consuming about 40-50 cups of coffee a day. But in that era, those cups were also very small. Given what he accomplished with his writings, it's safe to say that this *"black gold"* will definitely help us to become a high performing individual.

However, **caffeine works best for only some activities.** It may increase our attention span, the speed at which we work, prevent us from getting side-tracked, and may even benefit recall, but it's less likely to improve more complex cognitive functions.

Like with modafinil, you only get better at what you're already good at. You can't expand upon your existing cognitive limitations. The actual benefit you get is just more energy and alertness. In fact, it may actually harm tasks of higher executive functioning, such as creativity or problem solving, because large doses of caffeine may wire us up and cause shivers.

Use caffeine to rush through the repetitive activities that require a lot of micromanagement and aren't too difficult. This way you'll waste less time doing the small stuff and can free up more space for focusing on what's more important. With or without coffee depends on your own decision.

Drinking Coffee During Working Out

Once you take your first zip of the day, you can immediately feel your energy levels rising. This happens because your body will release more adrenaline and dopamine.

What ensues is lipolysis, which is the conversion of stored body fat into energy. However, the increased use of free fatty acids is reported to happen only in low carb/high fat diets[lxxxv]. Caffeine may be less useful on a high carb one[lxxxvi].

At the same time, coffee will still increase your metabolic rate and has other physical performance enhancing effects. Caffeine has a positive impact on muscular contraction and fatigue, which makes it a great tool for training.

Should You Drink Coffee Before or After a Workout?

When it comes to performance, then drinking a larger dose of caffeine 15-30 minutes earlier will yield some great results. Zipping on some beverage intra-workout is also viable. Even more, post-workout caffeine can also help to refuel muscles and increase fat burning[lxxxvii].

How to Drink Coffee Without Getting Addicted

As great as the benefits of caffeine are, we shouldn't overdose it by any means. Consuming it daily will increase our body's tolerance to it, which eventually leads to the receptors in our brain to becoming resistant to coffee. After some time, it stops working and we need a lot more to get the same effect.

Theodore Roosevelt drank a gallon of coffee a day. His son said that the president's mug was *"more on the side of a bathtub."*

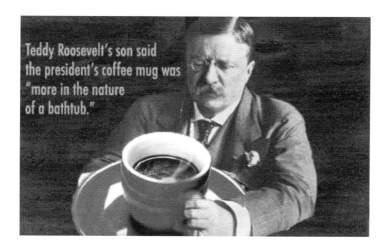

Teddy Roosevelt's son said the president's coffee mug was "more in the nature of a bathtub."

Even though the amounts consumed by Teddy and Voltaire might sound encouraging, don't try to drink as much as them.

Herein lies the point where people get addicted to coffee. They simply have developed a resistance towards caffeine and don't even feel like they've consumed it. To keep themselves awake, they reach out for another cup, crash and burn, and get another one, while getting stuck in the vicious cycle again.

To prevent that from happening, **you have to habitually cycle off caffeine.** For at least 1 week of the month you should allow your body's receptors to reset and become sensitive again.

Another option would be to drink coffee only on days where you most need it, say during a hard workout or while doing repetitive tasks.

This doesn't mean you can't drink coffee every day. You can. Simply swap out the caffeinated version with decaf. The taste is the same and you can get almost all of the benefits. If not the increased energy, then at least you'll still use it as an antioxidant and a mood enhancer.

What to Combine Coffee With

The effects of caffeine will also depend on what else is in your system at that time. Your metabolic type will already influence your rate of absorption but other nutrients will do so as well.

There are some benefits to consuming caffeine with glucose, which may improve cognition not seen with either alone[lxxxviii]. Additionally, grapefruit juice can keep caffeine levels in the bloodstream for longer[lxxxix]. If you're a slow oxidizer, then you may find adding these ingredients useful. Because we're on keto, this option isn't viable, unless you mask your drink with a lot of MCT or coconut oil.

If you're a fast oxidizer, then adding sugar will only hasten your downfall. You may get an immediate boost, but that short high will be followed by a steep low. To not crash and burn, you can add fat into the mix.

Dave Asprey's Bulletproof Coffee is probably the latest coffee drinking trend. Is it hype or does it actually work? Probably some of both. Adding butter to your cup of joe will definitely have some positive effects. It decreases the rate of absorption, gives you long-lasting energy, keeps you satiated for hours and tastes incredible. Whatever the case might be, you should try it. I also gave you my own Fatty Egg Yolk Coffee in Chapter Six.

Chapter Takeaway

- Don't drink coffee first thing in the morning or between 6 and 9 AM. Let your natural rise in cortisol wake you up and kickstart your day. If you feel tired, have a cold shower instead. Shocking...I know.

- Drink coffee between 9:30 and 11:30 AM or 1 and 2 PM.

- Don't drink large doses of caffeine after 4 PM.

- Use caffeine as a means of increasing the speed at which you cut through repetitive monotonous tasks.

- Use caffeine before working out to give you more energy and adrenaline.

- Cycle between caffeinated and decaf coffee. Once a month go at least 1 week without consuming caffeine.

Follow these principles and you'll set yourself up for long term success. Drink coffee effectively like a strategic genius and you'll eventually become one by reaping all of the benefits you get.

Conclusion

The World Is Yours

Do you think we're finished? Far from it – this is just the beginning to a much longer journey of self-experimentation and growth.

What I've done with this book is give you the ultimate guidebook on how to optimize your biology and shift it into its prime-primal state.

The knowledge written here is invaluable and highly effective. To be honest, once you become a fat burning beast and tap into your inner instinct, you'll become ever so powerful.

Doing Keto Fasting allows you to improve your health, enhance your cellular functioning, increase physical and cognitive performance and gives you access to abundant energy 24/7. As a result, everything you do will do gets better and more efficient.

Adapting to this way of eating can be difficult at times – whenever you feel exhausted, get nauseated by your keto breath or when you experience social pressure. But those are moments where your perseverance gets truly tested. If you stick to it, you'll eventually reach a point where you'll have circumvented all of the side-effects and will mostly reap the benefits.

With the abilities you possess you can accomplish great things. Once you become fat-adapted, it gets effortless for you to skip meals, never feel hungry, tired or lack energy. You'll be constantly tapped into your inner source of power and thus attaining an omnipotent state of vigor.

It has been a pleasure for me to write this book because I believe the information here will bring value to a lot of people. I've been testing, experimenting and tweaking my own nutrition for many years but I'm still not there yet. Far from it, this is just the beginning of a lifelong journey of self-discovery and growth.

If you're as big of an enthusiast about optimizing our own biology, improving on our psychology and general personal development, then you should definitely check out my blog at http://siimland.com/.

I also have a Facebook group for likeminded individuals who aspire to achieve great things while performing badass things. It's called the Body Mind Agoge and it comes with a FREE e-book that covers many other tools of greatness.

As a gift from me to you, get your free e-book at the end of this one and I'll see you on the other side.

Stay Empowered

Siim Land

FREE GIFT

Click the image above or the link below to get the **FREE** e-book

called Body Mind Agoge.

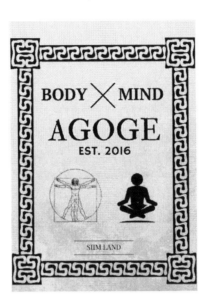

Or if you're on the paperback version, head over to

http://siimland.com/

Ultimate Keto Meal Plan

I've also created a 21 day ketogenic meal plan called Ultimate Keto, which will put ultimately into ketosis. It will help you to start a well-formulated ketogenic diet as a long term thing. Check it out.

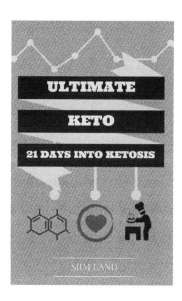

Click here to get Ultimate Keto!

Or If you're on the paperback, head over to siimland.com

I also offer high performance coaching about nutrition, training, mindset, habits, willpower and the like.

If you're interested, then contact me via e-mail:

siimlandd@gmail.com

More Books from the Author

Read more books in my Simple Keto series.

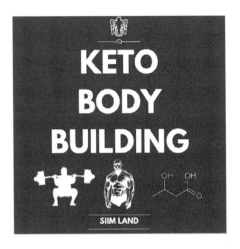

Keto Bodybuilding: Build Muscle, Burn Fat and Become a Beast on a Low Carb Ketogenic Diet

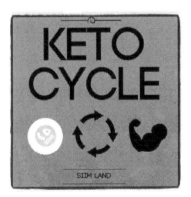

Keto Cycle the Cyclical Ketogenic Diet Book

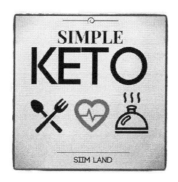

Simple Keto the Easiest Ketogenic Diet Book

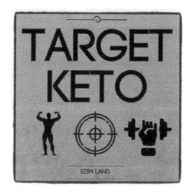

Target Keto the Targeted Ketogenic Diet Book

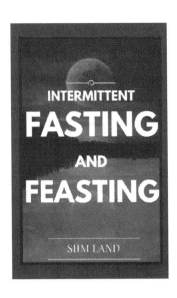

Intermittent Fasting and Feasting: Use Strategic Periods of

Undereating and Overfeeding

to Unleash the Most Powerful Anabolic Hormones of Your

Body

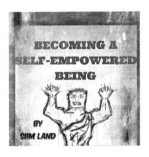

Becoming a Self Empowered Being

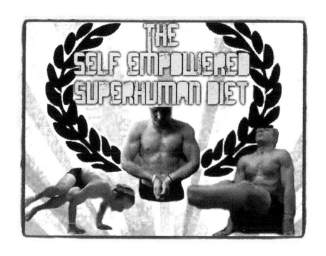

The Self Empowered Superhuman Diet

About the Author.

Hello, my name is Siim Land and I'm a holistic health practitioner, a fitness expert, an author and a self-empowered being. Ever since my childhood I've been engaged with personal development and self-actualization. As a kid, I made the decision of improving the state of mankind and transcending humanity towards the better. My journey has lead me on an Odyssey of body-mind-spirit, during which I've managed to develop and enhance every aspect of my being. My philosophy is based around achieving self-mastery and excellence first and foremost. What comes after that is the mission of empowering others to do the same. That's what I've dedicated my life to and am doing daily. To do that, I'm always trying to improve upon my own physiology, psychology and biology. I dream of a better world, in which mankind isn't separated from one another and is working towards reaching their truest potential.

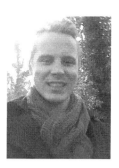

Contact me at my blog: http://siimland.com/contact

References

Here are all of the references to the studies mentioned in this book.

i Body composition and hormonal responses to a carbohydrate-restricted diet. Metabolism. 2002 Jul;51(7):864-70.

ii A high-fat, ketogenic diet induces a unique metabolic state in mice. Am J Physiol Endocrinol Metab. 2007 Jun;292(6):E1724-39.

iii What is an Essential Nutrient? Wikipedia.org

iv Endocrine Notes on Glucose Metabolism (PDF)

v Glycerol gluconeogenesis in fasting humans. Nutrition. 1995 Mar-Apr;11(2):149-53.

vi Low-carbohydrate nutrition and metabolism Am J Clin Nutr August 2007 vol. 86 no. 2 276-284

vii The Effects of a Ketogenic Diet on Exercise Metabolism and Physical Performance in Off-Road Cyclists Nutrients. 2014 Jul; 6(7): 2493–2508.

viii Nonenzymatic glucosylation and glucose-dependent cross-linking of protein. J Biol Chem. 1983 Aug 10;258(15):9406-12.

ix The AGE-receptor in the pathogenesis of diabetic complications. Diabetes Metab Res Rev. 2001 Nov-Dec;17(6):436-43.

x Advanced glycation end products. Dermatoendocrinol. 2012 Jul 1; 4(3): 259–270.

xi The effects of a low-carbohydrate ketogenic diet and a low-fat diet on mood, hunger, and other self-reported symptoms. Obesity (Silver Spring). 2007 Jan;15(1):182-7.

xii The National Cholesterol Education Program Diet vs a Diet Lower in Carbohydrates and Higher in Protein and Monounsaturated Fat. Arch Intern Med. 2004;164(19):2141-2146.

xiii HDL-subpopulation patterns in response to reductions in dietary total and saturated fat intakes in healthy subjects. Am J Clin Nutr December 1999

xiv Short-term effects of severe dietary carbohydrate-restriction advice in Type 2 diabetes--a randomized controlled trial. Diabet Med. 2006 Jan;23(1):15-20.

[xv] A low-carbohydrate, ketogenic diet to treat type 2 diabetes *Nutrition & Metabolism*2005**2**:34

[xvi] Metabolic syndrome and low-carbohydrate ketogenic diets in the medical school biochemistry curriculum Metab Syndr Relat Disord. 2003 Sep;1(3):189-97

[xvii]Metabolic characteristics of keto-adapted ultra-endurance runners. Metabolism Clinical and Experimental **March 2016**Volume 65, Issue 3, Pages 100–110

[xviii] Ketogenic diet does not affect strength performance in elite artistic gymnasts Journal of the International Society of Sports Nutrition20129:34

[xix] Grimm O. Addicted to food. Scientific American Mind 2007; 18(2):36-39

[xx] Owen OE, Felig P, Morgan AP, et al: Liver and kidney metabolism during prolonged starvation. J Clin Invest 1969 Mar; 48:574-583

[xxi] Heterothermy in growing king penguins. Nat Commun. 2011 Aug 16;2:435.

[xxii] https://en.wikipedia.org/wiki/Pareto_principle

[xxiii] Short-term fasting induces profound neuronal autophagy. Autophagy. 2010 Aug 16; 6(6): 702–710.

[xxiv] Alternate day calorie restriction improves clinical findings and reduces markers of oxidative stress and inflammation in overweight adults with moderate asthma. Free Radic Biol Med. 2007 Mar 1;42(5):665-74.

[xxv] Beneficial effects of intermittent fasting and caloric restriction on the cardiovascular and cerebrovascular systems. Journal of Nutritional Biology March 2005Volume 16, Issue 3, Pages 129–137=

[xxvi] Metabolic regulation of Sirtuins upon fasting and the implication for cancer. Curr Opin Oncol. 2013 Nov;25(6):630-6.

[xxvii] Tunstall RJ, et al. Fasting activates the gene expression of UCP3 independent of genes necessary for lipid transport and oxidation in skeletal muscle. Biochemical and Biophysical Research Communications 2002; 294:301-308

[xxviii] Enhanced thermogenic response to epinephrine after 48-h starvation in humans. Am J Physiol. 1990 Jan;258(1 Pt 2):R87-93.

[xxix] Resting energy expenditure in short-term starvation is increased as a result of an increase in serum norepinephrine. Am J Clin Nutr. 2000 Jun;71(6):1511-5.

[xxx] Alternate-day fasting in nonobese subjects: effects on body weight, body composition, and energy metabolism. Am J Clin Nutr. 2005 Jan;81(1):69-73.

[xxxi] Features of a successful therapeutic fast of 382 days' duration. Postgrad Med J. 1973 Mar; 49(569): 203–209.

[xxxii] Fasting enhances growth hormone secretion and amplifies the complex rhythms of growth hormone secretion in man. J Clin Invest. 1988 Apr; 81(4): 968–975.

[xxxiii] Merimee TJ, Fineberg SE: Growth hormone secretion in starvation: A reassessment. J Clin Endocrinol Metab 1974 Aug; 39:385-386

[xxxiv] Palmblad J, Levi L, Burger A, et al: Effects of total energy withdrawal (fasting) on the levels of growth hormone, thyrotropin, cortisol, adrenaline, noradrenaline, T4, T3, and rT3 in healthy males. Acta Med Scand 1977; 201:15-22

[xxxv] Roth J, Glick SM, Yalow RS, et al: Secretion of human growth hormone: Physiologic and experimental modification. Metabolism 1963 Jul; 12:577-579

Beck P, Koumans JT, Winterling CA, et al: Studies of insulin and growth hormone secretion in human obesity. J Lab Clin Med 1964 Oct; 64:654-667

[xxxvi] Nutritional regulation of the insulin-like growth factors. Endocr Rev. 1994 Feb;15(1):80-101.

[xxxvii] Practicality of Intermittent Fasting in Humans and its Effect on Oxidative Stress and Genes Related to Aging and Metabolism. Rejuvenation Research Volume: 18 Issue 2: April 21, 2015

[xxxviii] http://jn.nutrition.org/content/31/3/363.full.pdf

[xxxix] Dietary restriction increases the number of newly generated neural cells, and induces BDNF expression, in the dentate gyrus of rats. J Mol Neurosci. 2000 Oct;15(2):99-108.

[xl] Caloric restriction increases learning consolidation and facilitates synaptic plasticity through mechanisms dependent on NR2B subunits of the NMDA receptor. J Neurosci. 2007 Sep 19;27(38):10185-95.

[xli] Brain-derived neurotrophic factor as a regulator of systemic and brain energy metabolism and cardiovascular health. Ann N Y Acad Sci. 2012 Aug;1264:49-63

[xlii] Caloric restriction and intermittent fasting: Two potential diets for successful brain aging. Ageing Res Rev. 2006 Aug; 5(3): 332–353.

[xliii] Bloom WL: Fasting as an introduction to the treatment of obesity. Metabolism 1959 May; 8:214-220

[xliv] Williams RH (Ed): Textbook of Endocrinology-5th Ed. Philadelphia, WB Saunders, 1974

[xlv] The internal circadian clock increases hunger and appetite in the evening independent of food intake and other behaviors. Obesity (Silver Spring). 2013 Mar;21(3):421-3.

[xlvi] Grimm O. Addicted to food. Scientific American Mind 2007; 18(2):36-39

[xlvii] Ganley, R M. 1989. "Emotion and Eating in Obesity: A Review of the Literature." International Journal of Eating Disorders 8 (3): 343–361.

[xlviii] Neocortex Size, Group Size, and the Evolution of Language. Leslie C. Aiello and R. I. M. Dunbar Current Anthropology Vol. 34, No. 2 (Apr., 1993), pp. 184-193

[xlix] AMP kinase is required for mitochondrial biogenesis in skeletal muscle in response to chronic energy deprivation. PNAS vol. 99 no. 25 > Haihong Zong, 15983–15987

[l] Enhanced thermogenic response to epinephrine after 48-h starvation in humans. Am J Physiol. 1990 Jan;258(1 Pt 2):R87-93.

[li] Fasting enhances growth hormone secretion and amplifies the complex rhythms of growth hormone secretion in man. J Clin Invest. 1988 Apr; 81(4): 968–975.

[lii] Similar qualitative and quantitative changes of mitochondrial respiration following strength and endurance training in normoxia and hypoxia in sedentary humans. American Journal of Physiology. October 2011 Vol. 301 no. 4, R1078-R1087

[liii] Tunstall RJ, et al. Fasting activates the gene expression of UCP3 independent of genes necessary for lipid transport and oxidation in skeletal muscle. Biochemical and Biophysical Research Communications 2002; 294:301-308

[liv] Effects of moderate-intensity endurance and high-intensity intermittent training on anaerobic capacity and VO2max. Med Sci Sports Exerc. 1996 Oct;28(10):1327-30.

[lv] An acute bout of high-intensity interval training increases the nuclear abundance of PGC-1α and activates mitochondrial biogenesis in human skeletal muscle. Am J Physiol Regul Integr Comp Physiol. 2011 Jun;300(6):R1303-10.

[lvi] Resistance exercise enhances the molecular signaling of mitochondrial biogenesis induced by endurance exercise in human skeletal muscle. J Appl Physiol (1985). 2011 Nov;111(5):1335-44.

[lvii] http://Cold acclimation recruits human brown fat and increases nonshivering thermogenesis. J Clin Invest. 2013 Aug 1; 123(8): 3395–3403.www.ncbi.nlm.nih.gov/pmc/articles/PMC3726172/

[lviii] Brown adipose tissue: function and physiological significance. Physiol Rev. 2004 Jan;84(1):277-359.

[lix] Adapted cold shower as a potential treatment for depression. Med Hypotheses. 2008;70(5):995-1001. Epub 2007 Nov 13.

[lx] Adult hippocampal neurogenesis as target for the treatment of depression. CNS Neurol Disord Drug Targets. 2007 Jun;6(3):205-18.

[lxi] Human physiological responses to immersion into water of different temperatures. European Journal of Applied Physiology February 2000, Volume 81, Issue 5, pp 436–442

[lxii] Transient hypoxia stimulates mitochondrial biogenesis in brain subcortex by a neuronal nitric oxide synthase-dependent mechanism. J Neurosci. 2008 Feb 27;28(9):2015-24.

[lxiii] Hypoxia induces PGC-1α expression and mitochondrial biogenesis in the myocardium of TOF patients. Cell Research (2010) 20:676–687

[lxiv] Respiratory physiology: adaptations to high-level exercise. Br J Sports Med 2012;46:381-384

[lxv] The Expensive-Tissue Hypothesis: The Brain and the Digestive System in Human and Primate Evolution

[lxvi] The human metabolic response to chronic ketosis without caloric restriction: preservation of submaximal exercise capability with reduced carbohydrate oxidation.

[lxvii] Autophagy is required to maintain muscle mass. Cell Metab. 2009 Dec;10(6):507-15

[lxviii] Inflammation-Induced Alteration of Astrocyte Mitochondrial Dynamics Requires Autophagy for Mitochondrial Network Maintenance. Cell Metabolism Volume 18, Issue 6, p844–859, 3 December 2013

[lxix] Autophagy in the Pathogenesis of Disease. Cell Metabolism. Volume 132, Issue 1, p27–42, 11 January 2008=

[lxx] Bloom WL: Inhibition of salt excretion by carbohydrate. Arch Intern Med 1962 Jan; 109:80-86 48.

Veverbrants E, Arky RA: Effects of fasting and refeedingI. Studies on sodium, potassiulm and water excretion on a constant electrolyte and fluid intake. J Clin Endocrinol 1969 Jan; 29:55-62 49.

Botulter PR, Hoffman RS, Arky RA: Pattern of sodiuLm excretion accompanying starvation. Metabolism 1973 May; 22: 675-683

[lxxi] Chandra R, Liddle RA Cholecystokinin . Curr Opin Endocrinol Diabetes Obes. (2007)

Storr M, et al Endogenous CCK depresses contractile activity within the ascending myenteric reflex pathway of rat ileum . Neuropharmacology. (2003)

[lxxii] Geraedts MC, et al Direct induction of CCK and GLP-1 release from murine endocrine cells by intact dietary proteins . Mol Nutr Food Res. (2011)

[lxxiii] Soeters MR, et al Intermittent fasting does not affect whole-body glucose, lipid, or protein metabolism . Am J Clin Nutr. (2009)

Stote KS, *et al* A controlled trial of reduced meal frequency without caloric restriction in healthy, normal-weight, middle-aged adults . *Am J Clin Nutr*. (2007)

[lxxiv] Activation of autophagy is required for muscle homeostasis during physical exercise. Autophagy. Volume 7, 2011 - Issue 12. Pages 1405-1406

[lxxv] The neuroprotective effects of caffeine. Neurology August 7, 2007 vol. 69 no. 6 536-545

[lxxvi] Coffee consumption and risk of type 2 diabetes mellitus. The Lancet. Volume 360, No. 9344, p1477–1478, 9 November 2002

[lxxvii] Caffeine reduces the risk of Alzheimer's disease. https://biosingularity.wordpress.com/2006/09/15/caffeine-reduces-the-rish-of-alzheimers-disease/

[lxxviii] Association of Coffee and Caffeine Intake With the Risk of Parkinson Disease. JAMA. 2000;283(20):2674-2679

[lxxix] Adenosine, Adenosine Receptors and the Actions of Caffeine. BCPT. Volume 76, Issue 2

[lxxx] Modified-release hydrocortisone to provide circadian cortisol profiles. J Clin Endocrinol Metab. 2009 May;94(5):1548-54.

[lxxxi] Serum caffeine half-lives. Healthy subjects vs. patients having alcoholic hepatic disease. Am J Clin Pathol. 1980 Mar;73(3):390-3.

[lxxxii] Caffeine: A User's Guide to Getting Optimally Wired - http://scienceblogs.com/developingintelligence/2008/02/11/optimally-wired-a-caffeine-use/

[lxxxiii] Low-dose repeated caffeine administration for circadian-phase-dependent performance degradation during extended wakefulness. Sleep. 2004 May 1;27(3):374-81.

[lxxxiv] Human sleep, sleep loss and behaviour. Implications for the prefrontal cortex and psychiatric disorder. Br J Psychiatry. 1993 Mar;162:413-9.

[lxxxv] Influence of caffeine and carbohydrate feedings on endurance performance. Med Sci Sports. 1979 Spring;11(1):6-11.

[lxxxvi] A high carbohydrate diet negates the metabolic effects of caffeine during exercise. Med Sci Sports Exerc. 1987 Apr;19(2):100-5.

[lxxxvii] Post-Exercise Caffeine Helps Muscles Refuel - http://www.the-aps.org/mm/hp/audiences/public-press/archive/08/24.html

[lxxxviii] Cognitive and physiological effects of an "energy drink": an evaluation of the whole drink and of glucose, caffeine and herbal flavouring fractions. Psychopharmacology. November 2004, Volume 176, Issue 3, pp 320–330

[lxxxix] Inhibitory effect of grapefruit juice and its bitter principal, naringenin, on CYP1A2 dependent metabolism of caffeine in man. Br J Clin Pharmacol. 1993 Apr;35(4):431-6.

Made in the USA
San Bernardino, CA
16 March 2017